Sex, Love,

and

Chronic Illness

By Lucille Carlton

Enjoy!

Lucille Carlton

Library of Congress Catalog Card Number: 94-66888
ISBN: 0-9641712-0-1
Printed in the United States of America
10 9 8 7 6 5 4 3 2 1

Carlton, Lucille
    Sex, Love, and Chronic Illness

Cover design by: Paulette Livers Lambert

This book has been published through the generosity of the National Parkinson Foundation, Inc., Miami, Florida, for the benefit of all Parkinsonians and their caregivers.

This review appears in the May, 1994 edition of *American Health Magazine*. It was written by the former Editor-in-Chief of the Readers Digest, Mr. Kenneth 0. Gilmore.

LOVE AND PARKINSON'S DISEASE

After living with a man with Parkinson's disease for 16 years, Lucille Carlton shares her experiences in her book, *Sex, Love, and Chronic Illness* (National Parkinson Foundation, $13.95, to order call 800-327-4545; in Florida, 800-433-7022). The result; candid advice on how a couple can meet their sexual needs when one partner is physically limited. And this valuable information is packaged in a very readable book, mercifully free of neurological jargon.

Although Carlton focuses on the intimacy problems of couples when one person has Parkinson's, the information can certainly be applied to couples dealing with other physical handicaps. The author offers particular hope for those who fear their disabilities will keep them from enjoying sex.

Giving this account authenticity is the author's willingness to borrow from her own experiences. From bathtub to bed she provides a wealth of take-home material - information and ideas that can be used to help cope with daily living. For example, she explains the difficulty of persuading her husband to let her move to another bed because his restlessness was keeping her up at night. He feared the move would mark the end of their sexual relations. After assuring him that she would return to his bed every morning, she finally succeeded. (The book would have been even better if the author had cited more examples in which the husband is the caregiver.)

Carlton also describes how men who have become impotent can deal with that demoralizing problem. Be prepared for straight talk about masturbation and oral sex. And in a chapter for surviving spouses, the author counsels those who desire physical relationships. She presents readers with clear alternatives so that, free of guilt or shame, they can make their own decisions about how to satisfy their needs.

As one who has been in the clutches of Parkinson's for nearly a decade, I can say that this small book takes giant steps toward improving the quality of life of those afflicted - not to mention that of the caregivers who watch over us.

Kenneth O. Gilmore

I dedicate this book to my husband, who awakened passions deep within me and taught me the true meaning of love.

ACKNOWLEDGMENTS

With special thanks to Dr. Joseph Jankovic who suggested I write a book on sexuality; the National Parkinson Foundation for publishing the book; Emilio Alonso-Mendoza for his belief in my goals and for giving me the opportunity to help thousands of Parkinson families; Dr. Howard Hurtig, Dr. Carol Mackenzie and Gwyn Vernon for their confidence in my ability to bring off this project; Dr. Guila Glosser for her sensitive recommendations; and to The Mayo Clinic for technical information.

I extend my appreciation and gratitude to Dr. Matthew B. Stern, my mentor and No. 1 fan; Dr. Barney Dlin for his invaluable personal and professional opinions; Jane Wright, who shared ideas, dreams and philosophy with me; my daughter, Betsy Carlton, for our many honest and open discussions of sexuality; and to Phyllis Abrams, my unshockable friend.

A very special thanks to Susan Smith for her enthusiastic support and perceptive editing of the manuscript; Rita Verrilli, my perfectionist friend, for typing the manuscript; and to the Greater Philadelphia Parkinson Council for their generosity and support.

TABLE OF CONTENTS

FOREWORD

Matthew B. Stern, M.D., Director, The Graduate Hospital Parkinson's Disease and Movement Disorders Center and Associate Professor of Neurology, University of Pennsylvania

INTRODUCTION

RESOURCE DIRECTORY

FOREWORD

Despite the remarkable achievements in the treatment of Parkinson's disease in recent years, we remain largely ignorant of the causes of sexual function and dysfunction, and are therefore guilty of frequently dismissing one of the major reasons for despair in our patients. As a rule, neurologists are ill-equipped to deal with our patients' concerns regarding their sexuality. Combined with a natural reluctance by most couples to discuss sexuality with a virtual stranger, the Parkinsonian patient and partner are often left assuming that a satisfying sex life, like normal motoric function, is merely a vestige of a former life.

Understanding changes in sexual functioning that occur with neurologic impairment not only requires knowledge of normal physiology, but also necessitates some understanding of the complex psychosocial issues that affect the sexual response. Masters and Johnson have defined four phases of the "normal" sexual response cycle. These include the "Excitement phase" (nipple and penile erection, vaginal lubrication, flush), the "Plateau phase" (flush, muscle tension, increased heart and respiratory rate), "Orgasmic phase" (involuntary muscle contractions, ejaculation) and the "Resolution phase" (loss of flush and erection, resolution of increased heart and respiratory rate). The neurologic control of the various components of the sexual response cycle involves the entire nervous system, from brain to the small peripheral nerves that carry signals to and from the sex organs. Perhaps more importantly, the sexual response cycle is intimately associated with psychological factors. It is therefore difficult to distinguish between purely physical and psychological reasons for impaired sexual functioning. Our difficulties are further hampered by the psychosocial issues that accompany neurologic impairment (self-esteem, attractiveness, etc.). The result is the all too frequent exclusion of desirable sexual activity from our patients' lives and the avoidance of the subject of sexuality in the usual physician-patient interaction.

In Parkinson's disease, impairment in the sexual response may be the result of damage to specific areas in the brain or to dysfunction of the autonomic nervous system. Drugs used in the treatment of Parkinson's disease are also likely culprits in both inhibiting and increasing libido. Physical changes such as facial masking, drooling, hesitant speech and tremors affect the patient's self-esteem and diminish the sense of sexual attractiveness. Combined with slowness of movement and muscle rigidity, there are clear obstacles to entering even the initial (excitement) phase of the sexual response cycle. Nevertheless, there is no evidence that interest in sexuality declines either with age or in Parkinson's disease. A comprehensive approach to the treatment of patients with chronic illness, like Parkinson's disease, should therefore include helping patients develop alternative ways to enjoy pleasurable sexual relationships.

Lucille Carlton's frank discussions of love, sexuality, and chronic illness will indeed go a long way toward dispelling old notions regarding sexuality in elderly and impaired individuals. Told through the framework of her own wonderful relationship with her husband, Bob, who had Parkinson's disease for many years, Ms. Carlton has given us a much needed tool to promote more open discussions among health-care providers, patient and spouse and physician and patient. Her own roller-coaster ride through the many ups and downs of living with Parkinson's disease has given her a unique perspective which she, thankfully, has chosen to share with us. I have read "Sex, Love, and Chronic Illness" both as a neurologist treating patients with Parkinson's disease and as an individual aspiring to maintain my own loving relationship. Either way, this book is replete with useful information. Indeed, it is more about communication than sex, and how a loving and supportive relationship can overcome so many of the obstacles to intimacy that Parkinson's disease imposes.

Matthew B. Stern, M.D.
Director, The Graduate Hospital
Parkinson's Disease and Movement Disorders Center
and Associate Professor of Neurology
University of Pennsylvania

References:

1. Masters WH, Johnson VE. HUMAN SEXUAL RESPONSE. New York:

Bantam Books, 1966

INTRODUCTION

Sex has always been a difficult subject to discuss, and many people suffer in silence. Children avoid speaking about sex with their parents. Parents feel inadequate to discuss it with their children, their friends or even their partners. It is only in the last decade that senior citizens have begun to learn more–wanted to learn more–about this important part of their lives.

The reticence about sex began with our early lack of instruction in sexual matters. When we were young, women were told that husbands would instruct us, and this was all that we needed when we came to the marriage bed. Young men were admonished to be gentle and caring and not frighten their young brides. In today's world people are supposedly more sophisticated in their sexual knowledge. But many couples still find themselves ill-prepared to handle the sexual limitations imposed upon them by a chronic illness such as Parkinson's disease.

In fact, we still find that many people, old and young alike, are unable to communicate with one another or with professionals when it comes to talking about sexual fulfillment. They are also too embarrassed to ask for professional help. Because of time limitations in the doctor's office this issue is rarely raised. Women are often hesitant to initiate sex because they have been taught that it isn't ladylike to be the aggressor in the bedroom. This attitude often lasts throughout marriage. A particular problem arises when her spouse has a neurological illness such as Parkinson's disease and needs extra help for his slowed responses. He may be aroused emotionally, but his erection may be soft or short-lived.

Many factors enter into a woman's decision to avoid sexual intimacy with her Parkinsonian spouse. Some women feel that since child-bearing years are over, intercourse is no longer necessary. Some consider it an obligation, although their marriage is "solid." Every marriage, with or without health complications, is different; no two relationships are ever alike. We all respond in ways we think are correct for our situation at any given time.

We must also remember that there are wives who are burned out from waiting on an impaired spouse. The wife now does her chores and also assumes responsibilities that were formerly her husband's. She is depressed by his condition and worried about his decline and her uncertain future. She is usually exhausted physically and emotionally from lack of sleep. This certainly puts a damper on ardor.

In most situations, the male caregiver has a

more difficult role than the female caregiver. Women are natural nurturers, but this trait does not come easily to most men. The male caregiver must carefully balance the demands of his job with the new and powerful stress of role-reversal. He is now called upon to assume household chores, assist his partner with her clothing and help her maintain her attractive appearance. For a woman, little things such as squirming into pantyhose or dealing with a "bad hair day" can easily become a major undertaking. Small tasks soon escalate into giant frustrations and may be followed by depression for both partners. This can quickly impede sexual desires and abilities.

Some partners are turned off by the Parkinsonian's dyskinesia, strange body odor, profuse sweating or even drooling. When under stress, little things become exaggerated annoyances. Unfortunately, numerous wives do not know how to deal with sexual limitations. There is a narrow line between complete honesty and hurt feelings. Psychological scars come from too many put-downs. Each partner may feel a sense of rejection and will not be able to perform.

Many people are embarrassed by their sexual yearnings but are unable to communicate their needs, especially when they feel that the spouse would be unable to help. They do not want to give their partner additional stress but, on the other hand, they need separate beds or separate bedrooms. Then the opportunities to share sexual intimacy become fewer, and sexual activity is limited or nonexistent. When this occurs, some people are filled with guilt; others are relieved.

The male Parkinsonian may have sexuality problems. Many of the necessary medications have side effects that can cause impotence. Depression then sets in, eradicating desire for intimacy and increasing self-doubts. His feelings of masculinity have been stripped away. Parkinson's disease has robbed him of one more enormously important area of his life. He may already have had to surrender his driver's license and car keys, not to mention giving up a business or profession. Now this formerly independent man must face rejection of his sexual advances when he is unable to perform.

The side effects of medication, the wear and tear of aging, physical and emotional complications all contribute like dominoes to his impotence.

Perhaps, most agonizing of all, he finds virtually impossible to put into words the terror he feels. Aware of how much his spouse has already done for him, he hates to burden her further with his grief for the man he used to be–the man he'll never be again. It is a slow painful death of his spirit, leaving the shell of his former self. Oh, he still has sexual thoughts. No one can climb into his brain and obliterate them, thank goodness. But he desperately yearns for a true miracle–the restoration of his sexual drive.

All Parkinson couples share feelings of anger. This seems to be a universal emotion that demands acknowledgment. Some people try to bury these feelings and this usually makes matters worse. Others rage and rant but this only accelerates the level of stress in both partners. The anger is sometimes directed against the Parkinsonian. The caregiver feels: "How can you do this to me?" She lashes out in anger: "I agonize with you but I can only do so much. You must learn to do things for yourself and not depend on me all the time. You say that it's easier that way. For Whom? I resent having no time for myself. I am angry because I have to put your needs before my own."

Sometimes the anger is toward the caregiver, such as, "This disease strikes without discrimination. We both know that it is progressive. I didn't ask for it. I can't help my helplessness at times. Why can't you understand my frustrations, my limitations?"

Sometimes the anger is targeted at God: "I have led a good clean life and have tried to be a person who has helped my fellow man, so why do you punish me this way? Why me? What have I done to deserve this?"

Patients and caregivers often feel anger at themselves for being weak, for losing their temper, for losing control. They both have to realize that they are only human and must find a way to deal with life's adversities. There is never one correct answer, but there are ways to circumvent the frustration. The goal is to bring two loving partners the satisfaction of physical intimacy.

The purpose of the book is to educate and inspire creativity in handling the sexual needs of couples of all ages. It is written from the female point of view because my experience is as a wife/caregiver for sixteen challenging years. The information is also applicable to couples dealing with aging, cardiac, and cancer problems, with physiological disturbances, eating disorders, arthritis, rheumatoid diseases, bone/joint diseases and ostomies. I am confident that after reading this book you will find that the information also can apply to other problems.

Lucille Carlton,
Philadelphia, Pennsylvania

Doctor, please, I beg of you–
Can't you make me feel like new?
Stop the pain, ease my plight,
Banish every sleepless night.
Help me cope with ills unjust;
I've placed my life into your trust.

CHAPTER 1
IF YOU WANT TO KNOW,
YOU HAVE TO ASK

Dear Doctor_____ :

You and I are partners in handling my life with Parkinson's disease. I trust you and know that you will help me keep my life as normal as possible. You've examined me, medicated me, answered my questions honestly, and I've appreciated all that. You've given me pamphlets on nutrition, exercise, speech problems and other issues. But you have omitted giving me information about a most important part of my life–sex in my latter years.

The diagnosis of Parkinson's Disease was heartbreaking; it forced me into retirement and that was a blow. Then depression crept into the picture and hit me hard. Now my sexual problems have me reeling.

You haven't prepared me for this at all! We need something to help us keep our marriage on track. My wife feels guilty because she thinks she is no longer sexy enough to stimulate me. I feel guilty because I am depriving her of the happiness that she deserves. We want to satisfy each other but are met with frustration upon frustration. The atmosphere in our bedroom is uneasy and strained. Is it psychological? Is it medication? Is it Parkinson's? We NEED information on sexuality that we can share, and perhaps that will help keep our lines of communication open. We need printed and candid information which will help us avoid any embarrassment.

Our lives are not yet over! We have many obstacles to overcome, but a more realistic and happier sex life could make living with P.D. more bearable. I close my eyes and fantasize about the passions of long ago. But we need help now.

Sincerely,

_____

Can you identify with the person who wrote this letter? Do you have the urge to send it to your doctor? Couples in their sixties, seventies and eighties have had no preparation for dealing with their physical limitations and sexual dysfunction. Are sexual appetites supposed to disappear in your fifties? Our "golden years" become the most difficult and frustrating period of our lives. We must face the realization that we have to make the most of our present situation. We're expected to live life to the fullest in the time we have left on this earth. We notice signs of aging in our friends. We are able to accommodate the deaths of family members and our contemporaries, but we are most distressed when confronted by our own sexual dysfunction. It's a traumatic truth, and our problems can no longer be ignored. Questions arise:

How do we deal with this?

Do we try to solve the problem by ourselves?

To whom do we turn for help?

Can we adjust to our sexual limitations?

Many couples feel that their sexuality is a very personal matter and they decline to speak to anyone about it. They may even find it a difficult subject to discuss with each other. If this occurs, and discussion is avoided, it puts a severe strain on their relationship. The patient and the caregiver are already trying to deal with the stress of physical disability, the limitations imposed upon them by aging and the frustrations of daily togetherness known as retirement. Now sexual incompatibility becomes "the straw that broke the camel's back." It's never just one thing that pulls a relationship apart. It's many little things that accumulate and lead to dissension. It's painful to admit to sexual inadequacy in bed; the ego is fragile when it comes to sex. We may blame ourselves aloud, but we often harbor thoughts that the other person contributed more to our failures. At this point, an honest and open dialogue is imperative.

Self-help is an excellent starting point, and the

sooner you initiate it the better. My husband, for example, was an avid reader and learned everything he could find about Parkinson's disease. The same held true for his cardiac problems. He sought information on medications and their side effects, expected changes brought about by the progression of his symptoms, and anything that would enable him to cope with his declining abilities. He was always open to suggestions, and we were able to overcome the obstacles of his impaired health while still creatively satisfying our sexual needs.

Not everyone is that fortunate. A distraught woman phoned me recently on the recommendation of a mutual friend. She needed advice and didn't know where to turn. I did not know the woman, but I listened carefully. There were sexual problems within her marriage and she was certain that they were complicated by her Parkinson's disease. She had tried to bring this to her neurologist's attention, but she found that he never answered any of her questions of a sexual nature. She was saddened and frustrated by this experience and after several futile attempts to get answers finally gave up. Her questions should never have been ignored.

We must keep in mind that it takes time to develop a good doctor-patient relationship. We expect honest answers to our questions and we need a professional who will allay our fears. Health professionals are usually concerned with the patient's symptoms, progress and medications, and they earnestly try to keep within the time limits imposed upon them by their busy schedules.

I have found that if you send your doctor a very short note asking for time during your next appointment to discuss a special problem, the doctor will be most cooperative. If you do not wish your spouse to be present at this session, mention this in your letter. Some professionals feel ill-prepared to answer questions that may be outside their realm of expertise; others may shy away from questions of sexuality because the subject is so delicate. As much as we revere our doctors, they're only human. They cannot know everything or cure everything. We must be realistic in our expectations. If the doctor is unable to advise you on such a matter, he or she will be able to refer you to another authority such as a counselor, a nurse, gynecologist, urologist, social worker, psychiatrist or a psychologist. Sometimes the patient or caregiver needs to ask for specific help. Ask for any written material such as a book or brochure, or information about a support group or an organization that might send you literature on the subject. Remember, you are not alone, and the sexual problems of the aging or chronically ill should not be ignored.

In my conversations with health professionals and patients, I found that very few couples will consult the neurologist or health-care team about sexual matters. Men will sometimes broach the subject with a male doctor, but few females raise a question about sexuality when the neurologist is of the opposite gender. Couples should always ask questions about medications and understand the side effects associated with them.

When you have to consult a health professional it's important to remember that it usually takes several sessions with this person to become fully at ease. The professional is usually more comfortable handling a situation using clinical terminology. However, it is your right as a patient to ask for the explanation in simple layman's language, asking for greater detail or specifics if needed. Take notes if you are nervous, or bring a small hand-held tape recorder with you. Make certain that you question anything that is not clear to you. Prepare a written list of questions in order of their importance. Always be aware of time limitations, ask your questions in order of importance, and keep them brief. If you are more comfortable speaking with a professional of your same gender, request it. If you prefer a one-on-one conference, speak up and exclude your partner. You must be open and honest and not worry about hurt feelings. Arrange the session with consideration for your own psychological comfort level. Many therapists prefer to see the patient interact with the spouse so they can get a better assessment of the relationship. After that, you will be granted time alone for your session.

Some people cannot and will not talk to anyone, even a professional, about their intimate inadequacy. How do you balance your partner's negative reaction to your suggestion to seek help? Remember that it is your call and will affect your happiness for many years. If your mate refuses to go with you for counseling, go alone. The information and guidance you'll receive will help you deal with this distressing situation, and it may inject new life into your marriage. Slowly, gradually, let the knowledge you've acquired seep into your conversation and help you re-open communication about your sexual needs. The litany "we're too old for sex now" should be tossed away with yesteryear's relics. Repressed desires should not become a way of life.

I have no problems
It must be you!
Must I take the blame
For all YOU do?

CHAPTER 2
IS THERE A PROBLEM?

Dearest,

How do I begin? You call me Silent Sam and say I need to learn how to communicate, but when I bring up the subject of sex, you withdraw and become Silent Sally. It's something with which we have to deal, and we can't ignore it. We can't throw a blanket of silence over it and expect it to solve our problem. The sexuality thing is just a complication–another pesky challenge. I need your help. There–I said it! I swallowed my pride and made the first move. The next one is yours.

Let's not push this off until we go to bed–then tension will enter the picture. Can you sit down with me now? No blame–no shame? Promise?

Can you identify with this couple? Do words fail you when it comes to communicating your sexual needs and desires? You've been together for years and it's now time for an honest evaluation of an important part of your lives. How do you do this in a non-embarrassing, non-blaming way? Tackle it as you would any other problem.

1. Agree that there is a problem.

2. Identify the symptoms.
3. Ask how long the symptoms have bothered both of you.
4. Classify whether the problem is physical, emotional, or both.
5. Decide what annoys you the most and what frustrates you the least.
6. Prioritize! Put things in proper perspective: let go of the little things and tackle the larger picture.
7. Where do you turn for help? Can you help each other or do you need to talk with a professional?
8. Don't expect the problem to be resolved overnight. It will take time to turn it around. You must work at it to achieve the result you desire.

In my opinion, it is easier to communicate with each other if you sit side by side, touching. Your body language will say that you are not distancing yourselves from each other, and this is the most important step to agreeing. You are now willing to sit down and discuss the issue of ultimate closeness. Sometimes it's less painful to speak honestly if you don't have to make eye contact.

Start with the positive side and enumerate the things you always loved about sharing your life with your partner. Begin with generalities and work up to specifics. Give the other person time to speak as well, and at this point it is perfectly okay to interrupt each other. Think about what has just been said. Can one of you summarize the situation so far? What else can you add? Dig deeply into the GOOD things you can say about your relationship that you may have forgotten to mention. For example:

I loved the sweetness of your kisses.

I loved the tender way you stroked my beard.

I loved the soft way you looked at me.

I loved the way you flirted with me.

Sometimes you made me feel young again.

You made me feel special.

I loved the way you turned me on.

When you touched me I tingled.

When you put your head on my chest you made me feel protective.

I loved to feel the velvety smoothness of your skin.

I loved the way your laughter made me feel alive.

My fingers loved to trace the hollows of your body.

Remember the perfect rhythms we had? I could look into your eyes, catch your signals, and my body would respond to yours without breaking the tempo. Our lives used to be fun.

That's a beginning. Continue in this positive vein until you run out of wonderful memories, feelings you'd like to rekindle. By now you should be more mellow and ready to tackle the more difficult part of the conversation. What frustrates you in your relationship? Can it be remedied? How? Some sample comments:

When I want to make love, you're too tired.

What's more important–your clean kitchen or coming to bed with me?

I can't feel sexy just because you are in the mood.

You've turned into a mechanical lover - 30 seconds for this, 40 seconds for that.

You lie there like a lifeless lump.

When you enter me, it hurts.

Don't pull at me–I'm sensitive.

I need more foreplay.

I need to be held and caressed after I climax, but you just roll over and snore.

I can't stand all these distractions. They break my mood.

Can you identify with any of the above? I'm certain you can easily add to this list.

When things bothered me and I found it difficult or embarrassing to find the right words, my husband would say, "Just blurt it out. Don't worry about words or hurt feelings. Blurt it out; we'll sort it out after that." This always worked for us. If he needed to "get something out of his system" (his favorite expression) he, too, would warn me and then blurt it out. It's really much simpler this way. Then we went at it piece by piece, sentence by sentence, until we each understood how to handle the sticky problem.

At this point it's usually best to stop and sit quietly holding each other, letting the past dialogue slowly seep in. You've reached a point of saturation, it's true. But you have also given your partner a chance to regroup. You've allowed time for the ideas to make an impression and now you must turn your thoughts to practical ways to cope with the problems. You and your partner have taken the first constructive steps toward improving your lines of sexual communication.

I believe that honesty is the foundation of a good relationship. Look inside yourself and make an honest assessment of what you have said or done as well as your underlying motives for doing so. We're all selfish to some extent. At times our words have hurt those we love, but no one is perfect. Words spoken in anger can never be retracted, no matter how many apologies are offered. Sometimes it's a matter of pride, sometimes it's merely stubbornness, but most people are unable to make the first move toward reconciliation.

It's unhealthy in a relationship to harbor negative thoughts, which feed upon themselves and turn an insignificant misunderstanding into a major hassle. Some of us clam up and nurse the resentment that gnaws at us. Others are able to put hurt feelings into words, and this hastens the resolution of any problem.

In our marriage we often preferred the written word. When I was upset, tears of frustration got in the way of an explanation or an apology.

I have always been troubled by lengthy bouts of laryngitis. Bob hated the virus because it lasted from several days to several weeks. He had a hearing problem and my whispers were difficult for him to understand. This was also a time of low energy for me and total frustration for both of us.

The doctor warned me not to whisper. Consequently, I resorted to writing notes. There were scraps of paper bearing scribbled messages all over our apartment. Bob kept his comments to a minimum because he knew it frustrated me to be unable to answer him. I felt like I was living in a vacuum or in a chamber of silence. I'm a gregarious person and need sound. I devised a hand signal that meant talk to me but Bob soon tired of seeing me flash this signal to him countless times a day. "What more can I say to you?" he'd ask. "I'll be glad when her voice returns" was mumbled under his breath.

One particularly bad day I scribbled on my tablet, "Can't you talk to me? I do so much for YOU all of the time I do everything but breathe for you. You expect so much of me. It's Lu, do this and Lu, do that. I'm your wife and not your slave." I ripped the page from the pad and shoved it at him and marched out of the room. My defenses were down. I was ill, irritable and terribly frustrated. I needed space and time to soothe my injured feelings. An hour later when I emerged from the bedroom I heard the clickety-clack of typewriter keys. Bob looked up and smiled and said, "I'm typing this letter so you won't be frustrated by my chicken-scratch handwriting." He typed slowly, using the hunt-and-peck system, but before long he took me in his arms and presented me with the following letter:

Dearest,

What do you do for me? Literally everything that can be done. You are my cook, housekeeper, secretary and social director. You are my nurse and my chauffeur, my reminder and my helpmate. You are my friend and my lover as well as the best wife a man could ask for! You are the support system and shelter I need to help keep me on an even keel. You comfort me and I rely on you to keep me moving through the days

and nights.

I hate to add to your worries but sometimes I think you worry more than you need to. I don't blame you for being peevish sometimes, but you let too many small things get to you that you should shrug off. I know it drives you up a wall when I don't talk to you and you say talk to me, but I don't have a fund of small-talk. I try not to prolong discussions of my Parkinson's condition, as this would give you only more to worry about. I try to be helpful around the apartment but I am forgetful and not as precise as you would like me to be. I'm sorry. I do try to lessen your burden as much as possible.

I hate to see you lose your voice, for my sake as well as yours. I have difficulty making out what you are saying, so I hesitate to start up with any extra conversations.

I do love you with all my heart, but I fail to show it at times. You are the sun in my galaxy and all that I am revolves around you.

Lu, I love you

My anger and frustration melted with each sentence that I read. His kisses soothed me, his arms comforted me, and the spoken word lost its importance.

Bob loved to browse in card shops and find

printed sentiments that expressed his feelings or concerns. The cards weren't only for holidays or special occasions, but for any time that my sentimental husband wanted to convey a special message to me. Some cards were funny, some were romantic.

Sometimes a message would be scribbled on a scrap of paper and placed upon my pillow in the morning to be found when I made the bed. The previous evening's intimacies had inspired this message:

Dearest,

The flesh may be weakened but the desire and love remain vigorous.

Love you.

That little note put both of us in a mellow and appreciative mood the entire day. Aches and pains and disabilities were of little importance. We were like hand-holding youngsters once more.

Bob was not the only one to communicate in this way, solving problem areas in our marriage. I gave him an envelope marked:

RX: Please read and reread when I get you down, or you can't understand me, or I nag you too much.

The enclosed letter read:

Dearest,

I tell you of my love each day of our lives, but it is typical of me to repeat myself. Your love has been the most wonderful gift of my life. I don't know what I've ever done to deserve it, but I am grateful God has rewarded me this way. I wish my love could envelop you and protect you from hurt, be it mental or physical. My love for you will always be there–and even when I'm gone it will be there to comfort you.

We need each other, Bob dear, and we must take care of one another so that we can share this unique happiness for many years to come.

I thank you, darling, for your patience with me when I have my ups and downs and can't explain them. I thank you for your encouragement when I attempt any creative project. I thank you for your understanding when I am terrified over little things. I thank you for your wisdom and your calm support when I am devastated by worry. I thank you for the beautiful life you have given me.

But most of all, darling, I thank you for your love and you.

Forever yours,
LU

Some problems are minor, some are of greater importance. Both partners must understand that their ever-present need for touching, caring and love may be a crucial factor in coping with chronic illness. Patience, honesty and communication are also vital ingredients for the proper mix.

"Talk to me!" he heard her say.
Said he, "I thought we did that
yesterday."

CHAPTER 3
TALK TO ME

Do you find yourself making excuses each night?
"Go to bed, dear. I have just a few more chapters to read. I may even finish this book tonight, so don't wait up for me."

or

"I really must get this paperwork completed. Go to bed without me. I'll be up later."

or

"I'm bushed and I'm going to bed early. Take your time coming to bed–and please don't wake me."

or

"You look tired. Go to bed without me. There's a TV program I want to see but it's a late one. I'll tell you about it tomorrow."

or

"I have to figure out this computer problem or else I won't be able to fall asleep. I have too much on my mind right now. Go to sleep without me."

or

"My muscle rigidity is too great. I'll go to bed when I'm ready, and not before. I won't wake you."

The truth of the matter is that you are probably trying to avoid the issue of sex. You don't want your body touched, only to be frustrated. You just want to be left alone. But you don't know how to say this to your spouse. What words could adequately express your feelings? Is it just for this night? For a few weeks? Forever? You are on an emotional roller-coaster anyway, and in your mind, sex or the lack of it, is just another complication. You do not wish to deal with it!

Try to envision the following scenario:

The Parkinsonian and his wife prepare for bed, and before they slip under the covers he reaches out for her.

Husband: "Do you want to?"

Wife: (silence)

Husband: "Try again?"

Wife: "Nooo, I don't think so."

Husband: "I'm okay now, really I am."

Wife: "I'd rather not."

Husband: "Don't say I didn't ask."

Wife: "It's okay with me if you never ask."

They slip under the covers, he on his side of the bed, she on hers, as far apart as they can be. He is crushed, dejected, hurt. He thinks, "With

Parkinson's I have my down times and I have my good times. Why can't she help me take advantage of my 'up' periods? Is that asking too much? Sex was always a wonderful part of our lives. It brought us so close to each other. Now there's a great chasm dividing us–just one more area where we're distancing ourselves. This disease is no picnic, but I can handle it. All I ask is some sign of love and support."

His wife is in bed, eyes shut, but with tears near the surface. She thinks "How often do we need to go through this? I love him. I just have no desire to have sex with him. I hate it when he looks like a wounded puppy, but doing nothing is better than the unfulfilled promise of the ultimate sexual experience. I get too frustrated and then lose my cool, and I can't handle it. We'll have to settle this thing once and for all. There's always TOMORROW–we'll talk tomorrow–MAYBE."

We were at a family gathering when a relative took my husband aside and told him he wanted advice. "Man-to-man stuff," he said. "I need your input as one Parkinsonian to another. I'm stymied, and don't know where to turn." "When I touch Edith I never get a response. It's as if she's a rag doll lying there or a statue. There's absolutely no movement on her part. I can't do it all by myself. I need some encouragement, some sign that there's life under my hand. When I ask her what's going on she just tells me that she's interested, but she's not aroused. In that mood who could succeed? I remind her that when we were younger I could have an erection immediately just by looking at her naked body, but now it takes longer. I need a little cooperation, a little patience and understanding. We have to take advantage of an erection quickly, because it doesn't last too long these days.

"She usually glares at me, and in icy tones informs me that she knows all about it and is tired of my complaints. Her refrain is always the same: 'Hold me if you must, but let me get some sleep. TONIGHT'S NOT THE NIGHT - that's all.'"

"Bob, I'm not a mind reader I just wish Edith would tell me what she wants."

Have you been able to discuss this with your partner? A discussion of sex involves intimate feelings. Many people shrink from doing this even with their closest loved one, because they fear the other person's reaction to what's being said. To reveal your innermost emotions is to bare your soul. Sexual dysfunction is often something that we cannot control yet it fills us with shame, so we decline to discuss it. The old saying "Use it or lose it" is often true. The longer you abstain from sex the more difficult it is to recapture the ability to perform, and the sexual responses have to be re-educated. Sexual frustrations are very stressful for both partners. You must talk about the problem calmly without blaming anyone. The key is NO BLAME because sexual dysfunction and decreased desire are not chosen responses. If you feel that you are unable to handle this emotionally charged issue, speaking with a therapist or counselor will often help.

It's really no one's business what occurs in the privacy of your bedroom(s). You and your partner need to decide jointly what best suits your needs, your abilities and your relationship, without regard to "what others might think" if they knew. A caregiver friend said that bedtime was her favorite time "for herself." She told me that they usually retired early in the evening because her husband's Parkinsonism kept him awake much of the night. She said she always tucked Ed into bed with a good-night kiss planted on his shiny bald head, and then went to her own room to meditate. After this routine, she turned her bedside radio to soft music, and then read her book until her eyelids grew heavy. It was a time of relaxation, a time of renewal, and a time that was her special escape from their daily problems.

If your partnership is comfortable with little or no sexual activity, you must find another way to communicate your love for each other on a daily basis, for this is needed to take up the void. Human beings need to be kissed, to be touched and hugged. It's also comforting to have your shoulder patted, your hand held or your back or neck gently rubbed. It is reassuring to catch a smile, a wink or a silent kiss that is sent your way across the room. They're all signals that your spouse cares. Declarations of love are sometimes verbal and sometimes non-verbal in nature. A simple suggestion delivered with a smile and accepted with a nod, such as:

> **"I'll help you out of your chair, dear, if you'll join me in the kitchen for our bedtime snack." translates to:**

> **"We're here to help each other. I care enough to share some goodies with you before going to bed, and they're your favorites. Our little routines are not boring I look forward to our affectionate banter."**

A homey little routine such as this brings a sense of comfort and security to people who have shared many years.

I always enjoyed curling up on the sofa with my head resting upon my husband's lap. He may have been reading a book at the time, or watching a program on television, but he'd stop now and then and run his fingers through my hair. It was a cozy and reassuring silence for both of us, but it spoke volumes.

Many couples are comfortable merely sharing tasks and ideas, and handling the ups and downs of daily living. Sex is no longer a priority, and they just want to enjoy the blessed companionship of living together. It's okay to say, "I truly love you and love the caring person that you have always been. We've shared so many years of togetherness, and I treasure that. While I'm happy to be your helpmate, I am less enthusiastic about our sex life. At this point, I would be content with a loving closeness, but I'd like to leave the sexual part of our lives to past memories. I no longer want sex, but I do crave love, and love is the glue that will continue to keep our marriage together."

Sex isn't for everyone. It's your choice. Just be comfortable with your decision, together.

Men think women are the weaker sex,
Emotional and quite complex.
Women, on the other hand,
Are learning NOW to take a stand.

CHAPTER 4
WOMEN'S WOES

Have you ever heard your spouse say, "Every time I think I understand you I find that I don't"? Men feel that women are complex beings who never say what they mean. Women will fuss about the little things, but will be silent over the underlying cause for the emotional upset. My husband would say that he wasn't a mind reader, but I would tell him that he just wasn't tuned in to my needs. What is obvious to a woman may be an unknown factor to her spouse. In the early years of marriage, husbands grumble, "That time of the month again—heaven help us." In midlife they shake their heads and complain, "Menopause," and in their golden years they merely throw up their hands and declare, "I guess I'll go to the grave never understanding women and their moods!"

In our youth most of us struggled each month with the discomfort of menstruation. There was bloating from water retention, cramps and emotional turmoil. Some girls had heavy blood-flow and they'd say that they were "flooding." The terminology was bizarre; menstruation was also known as "the period, the curse, or falling off the roof" (I never could make sense of the latter.) Of course there were young women who were blessed with a 28-day cycle and who were free of pain. At the other extreme were young women whose flow lasted several weeks and whose periods were fewer in number. Women half-joked that they could always count on their menstrual period to arrive in time to ruin plans for holidays, vacations or special events. Such was life.

Menopause takes place between the ages of 35 and 55. With the cessation of menstruation, various reactions occur: Some females mourn the loss of their reproductive ability while others view menopause as a gift that takes away the "monthly mopes." The majority of women are grateful to be free from worry about pregnancy. This brings about a more relaxed attitude toward intercourse. Couples look forward to intimacy with nothing artificial between them. This is happiness.

Sometimes the happiness is short-lived because menopause, due to a decrease in the estrogen level, brings about changes in the woman's body. Her sex organs decrease in size and elasticity. A menopausal woman experiences embarrassing hot flashes and flushes. All of a sudden her color will deepen to a red blush, she'll break into a sweat, and perspiration drips from her. At times the bedsheets and/or her nightgown have to be changed during the night because they are drenched with perspiration. Hot flashes occur at any time and have nothing to do with room temperature or time of year.

Accompanying these symptoms are mood swings and episodes of super-sensitivity and tears. She feels bloated, unattractive, constantly tired, and has a lowered or negative interest in sex. The jokes about "Not tonight, dear, I have a headache," are really based upon truth. Menopausal women are subject to headaches, neckaches and fatigue.

Menopause is a normal part of a woman's life-cycle. During this time her ovaries stop producing estrogen. Estrogen is a hormone that plays an important role in the reproductive system, helps bones remain strong and protects against heart attacks. When estrogen levels are low, changes in the vagina and urinary tract take place, and bone loss may also occur. The older woman's bones slowly lose calcium and protein. Bones become brittle and break easily.

Female sex organs change in size and shape. Now the depth and diameter of the vagina is reduced. It actually narrows and becomes shorter. Although the vagina loses some of its elasticity it will still be able to stretch enough to accommodate the penis. The labia, or outer lips of the vagina, will sag and lose muscle tone. The clitoris will also decrease in size but it will still retain its sensitivity. The hood that protects the clitoris thins with age. Love-play of the clitoris can be delightfully exciting at the beginning, but too much pressure or prolonged fondling can become painful after a while. The woman's bladder and urethra are now less protected and they may become irritated during intercourse.

Hormone replacement therapy can be used successfully but it is not for everyone. It has risks that must be assessed by the doctor and the patient. Many doctors will advise a woman to take progesterone as well as estrogen because it is thought to lower the risk of endometrial cancer. However, it is best to allow YOUR gynecologist to advise you about the need for hormone replacement. Everyone's situation is different. Many women report that they feel healthier and more energetic when taking hormones. Estrogen replacement can be found in pill form, skin patches, suppositories or vaginal creams. The latter prevent vaginal dryness, but they do not work as well on the other menopausal symptoms.

Women practitioners are now making inroads in the once male-dominated field of gynecology. Older women are learning new attitudes about their bodies from their younger "sisters" and they're seeking gynecologists of their own gender, feeling that only a woman can understand the emotional turbulence women experience during menopause and post-menopausal years.

Women hate lying on the examining table, quivering legs spread apart, and feet jammed into the stirrups. Thoughts of the cold speculum being pushed into the vagina by a male physician make some women grit their teeth. Patients take deep breaths and endure the uncomfortable probing and clinical examination. They only wish to get off the table as quickly as possible, and not lie there resenting the invasion of privacy. At the doctor-patient conference that follows the examination, questions and answers are usually brief. Many women are uncomfortable exposing their concerns about this very private part of their lives.

At lunch one day I joined a group of women who were animatedly discussing this subject. Rita said, "You know how I always put off going to the gynecologist? Well, I finally made an appointment with a woman doctor and it made all the difference in the world to me. I could open up to her and she understood my miserable night-sweats and my tears. In fact, I cried when I told her about my husband's frustration with me, and for once I wasn't ashamed of my tears. I'm moody and I am no longer as interested in sex as I've been in the past, and that's a bone of contention in my marriage. Woman to woman, she understood me and explained what was happening to my emotions and the changes taking place within my body. When my appointment was over, I hugged her and walked out feeling better about myself than I had in a long time." Every woman in the group had a story to tell. They commiserated with one another; and a few suggested self-help books that had proved valuable.

Another frustration for the older woman is her lack of vaginal lubrication. An application of K-Y jelly to the vaginal area assists the natural secretions, easing penetration by the penis; thus, pain caused by friction is avoided. It takes older women longer to lubricate, just as it takes older men longer to have an erection.

A common problem with women is stress-incontinence. This is the seepage of urine when a woman coughs, sneezes, laughs or exerts herself. Women who have given birth several times will identify with this problem. The Kegel exercises, described at the end of this chapter, will help build up the muscles that support the bladder. Consult your doctor for further information if other methods are needed to rectify your situation. It helps to empty your bladder frequently. Although pantyliners do not cure anything, they save embarrassment when an accidental spill occurs. Before you prepare for physical intimacy make certain that your bladder is emptied. Some women discharge a small amount of urine at the height of arousal. It is nothing to be ashamed of. Discuss this with your partner and place a clean soft towel on the bed under your hips. It should not interfere with your pleasure, and your partner probably will not be turned off by this. Make light of it. Your attitude will affect his attitude.

I've spoken with Parkinsonian women who have a variety of reactions to questions about sexual ability. I asked if dyskinesia interfered with their love life. Helen told me that sex is best for her and her husband when she is OFF (For a Parkinsonian OFF means that the medication is losing effectiveness, and this is often described as end-of-dose-letdown; ON occurs when the medication is working at peak efficiency). They've devised a unique position that is best for their situation, and they've found happiness in this discovery. Other female Parkinsonians have told me that they must wait until they're ON, enabling them to be more relaxed and agile enough for physical activity. Parkinsonism does not interfere with desire.

A Parkinson friend confided that her husband complained that she "never looked interested" so he hesitated to broach the subject of sex. He had to be educated about the PARKINSON MASK, which prevents the facial muscles from displaying emotions. "I really am interested in sex" she said, "but not as often as he is. He always wants it at bedtime, and that's when my symptoms are at their worst." I asked her who initiates sex in their marriage and I was not the least bit surprised to learn that her husband was the one to suggest it. As much as she wanted sexual intimacy during her ON time, she never felt it was ladylike to speak up for it.

She kept waiting and hoping. They both needed to be taught that there is no special timetable for making love. Communication is the key.

Every woman, young or old, needs to feel that she is desired. It's up to her to agree to intimacy or to decline the invitation. Perhaps all she desires at that particular time is some cuddling and kissing, a bit of tenderness. This is often a preliminary that escalates to more intense lovemaking. Levels of arousal can be intensified rather rapidly.

There are many females who are conditioned to wait for their partner to initiate sex. But nothing is as exciting as a woman's invitation to "Come into the bedroom with me. Today I'll be your dessert." If that's not your style, that's okay. Put it in your own words, but let your actions accompany your invitation. Your partner will be singing your praises as he joins you. It does not matter who initiates sex. A creative invitation becomes a turn-on for both sexes.

KEGEL EXERCISES

Millions of women experience stress incontinence, which causes urinary leakage when they cough or sneeze. In 1952, Dr. Arnold Kegel devised exercises to help women with pelvic muscle problems. The exercises strengthen the pubococcygeus muscle (called the PC) and improve bladder control. The PC muscle allows you to interrupt urinary flow or to push out those last drops of urine.

The easiest way to locate the PC muscle is to place your finger inside your vagina and squeeze After doing this several times you will be able to identify the area without the use of your finger. When squeezing or contracting the muscle, be gentle and don't strain.

1. After you have located the PC, squeeze and hold for a count of 5. Then relax for the same length of time. Don't rush it. Relaxing the muscle is just as important as squeezing.
2. Gradually increase the time until you can do the exercise 10 or 15 times a session.
3. Do the exercises three times daily.
4. Build your muscle strength slowly and do not expect immediate results. You should see improvement in 3 to 4 weeks.

The beauty of this exercise is that it can be

done anywhere and at any time. No one will be able to know that you are exercising this muscle. It's easy to do–it just needs practice.

He won't behave—
My recalcitrant Knave!

CHAPTER 5
THE FEAR OF IMPOTENCE

Impotence is a condition that men fear. It can affect them at any age or any time. Younger men panic and worry about their testosterone levels. Older men curse it and believe that their last shred of masculinity has been stripped away. Men of all ages who are faced with impotence feel angry, depressed and frustrated. They are pulled in two directions: to speak or not to speak is a question that looms large. Men who are impotent are afraid to talk about it, yet they desperately need information, help and support.

Impotence is the temporary or permanent inability to have an erection or maintain it long enough to have successful sexual intercourse. It can be caused by psychological factors, illness or medications. It is said that the penis is the barometer of a man's feelings. Fatigue, stress and drug and alcohol abuse can add to the problem. Anxiety and fear can diminish a man's sexual ability.

I visited an impotence clinic to obtain literature on the subject. The waiting room was large and bright with chairs arranged in conversational groupings. When I entered the room, no one looked up. Each man had seated himself as far away from the others as possible. Each person appeared completely engrossed in a newspaper, magazine or book. No one exchanged words or glances. It was as if a subliminal message had been communicated: **I don't want to talk about it. I know why I'm here and I guess you're here for the same reason. Don't ask me questions!**

An uneasy silence in the room was broken by the rustling newspaper pages being turned. The receptionist handed me brochures the doctor had gathered for me. As I departed, I saw that all the men made it a point not to notice who was entering the office or leaving. The message was clear: Don't invade my space!

My husband was an Army captain during the Korean War. Several months before his discharge from the service, he began having erectile difficulties. He was young, the father of two small children, and had never before experienced failure to perform. Bob was embarrassed and angry. I was disappointed and shared his frustration, but I was determined to try to understand the situation.

I discreetly spoke with the ranking nurse on the Post, figuring she would have medical knowledge. I didn't want to confer with any doctor there because most of them were our friends and Bob would not have wanted any of them to know he was having sexual problems. I explained to Anne that our conversation had to be confidential. She listened to my pleas for information and said, "Nothing to worry about. That's **just men**. They'll say or do anything to keep from using contraception. They'll say it keeps them from performing or that they do better without it. Your husband's like the rest of them. Men will do anything to get their own way."

I was horrified and left her office in a daze. I was convinced that she was wrong. She didn't know. Bob wasn't like that! I was furious. Why did I break our silence? I was ashamed that I had violated our privacy, and I hoped that my husband would forgive me.

When Bob got off duty that night I confessed that I had spoken about our sexual difficulties. I meant well. I thought that I was reaching out for help. At first my husband was angry. Then he simmered down and said that he understood my frustration with his impotence. Bob dried my tears, and with false bravado told me that it was probably temporary. He promised that as soon as he was discharged from the Army he'd make an appointment with a urologist or an endocrinologist. In the meantime he asked for more patience on my part.

He followed through on his promise to seek medical assistance. He was told that his impotence was caused by worry about returning to civilian life, reopening his veterinary hospital and regaining his former clients, and being able to provide for his family during the interim. The endocrinologist gave him medication to improve his testosterone level and assured him that this was only a temporary inconvenience.

Once the problem was addressed it didn't take long before Bob's sexual performance improved. This happened when he was thirty, but the memory of it lingered throughout his lifetime. Years later, Bob declared that impotence would never again get him down because he was aware of other options to achieve sexual gratification.

Every man experiences an erectile failure at some time. It can be triggered by the inopportune ringing of the telephone, a knock at the door, an inappropriate comment, an unresponsive partner, or a cry of pain instead of pleasure. Erections are sensitive to distractions. Younger men can usually regain an erection rapidly. Older men have a longer refractory period.

Have you ever said the spirit is willing but the flesh is weak? Have you ever been chastised with "You're no youngster anymore. What do you expect at your age? So you're impotent–learn to live with it."

Impotence can shatter a man's self-confidence. Concern about sexual performance leads to stress and pressure to perform, which leads to an inability to perform. On and on it goes, with frustration, anger or depression feeding into the mix. To disrupt the vicious cycle, some intervention is necessary. I suggest that, instead of being angry and depressed, you consult your family physician and ask for a referral to a specialist.

The first step is to make certain that there is no physical cause for your impotence. The physician will take a medical history as well as a psychological and sexual history. You'll be asked questions pertaining to your early-morning erections and how long it takes to achieve an erection. There will be questions about your lifestyle, your cholesterol and your weight. The doctor will want to know if you've had surgery or physical problems. He or she will want to know how you feel about yourself and your interactions with your partner.

Prescription drugs or over-the-counter medications may contribute to your problem, or you may have a simple hormonal imbalance. Many Parkinson medications, anti-hypertensive drugs, tranquilizers and anti-depressants can cause erectile dysfunction as a side effect. Speak to your physician about your medications. The dosage may need to be changed, or you may need to be switched to another medication that will have no adverse effects upon your libido.

Depression is a prominent cause of a lowered

or nonexistent sex drive. It sometimes accompanies an illness and/or aging. On occasion, serious illness may trigger the fear of death. Poor sexual performance for physical or psychological reasons may also activate a man's fears about aging and mortality, followed by self-inflicted derision, anger and resentment. These are nonproductive reactions that may lead to chronic or acute clinical depression. Despondency leads to impotence, which in turn increases depression.

Do not wallow in self-pity. Urologists, psychologists, endocrinologists, psychiatrists, sex therapists or counselors are all there to offer help and they may be able to provide remedies that will enhance your sex life. If not, press for alternatives that may improve this condition. Enlist a professional's help immediately.

I'm feeling down,
Seems nothing's right.
I try to hide
My chilling fright.
>*I've seen her tears*
>*And we both know*
>*Depression follows*
>*Where e'er we go.*

CHAPTER 6
WHO'S DEPRESSED?

We had known for several years that Bob definitely had Parkinson's disease. This was devastating but we were determined to get through each day as best we could. Bob was especially concerned that he might not be able to keep up with the heavy demands of his veterinary practice while also combating the unrelenting progression of Parkinson's.

I knew that Bob had been working longer hours, driving himself as if someone had a whip in his back. He'd fall into bed each night too exhausted to sleep. But it wasn't until I saw his tears that I finally realized that we faced a serious problem. Why had I not noticed this before? I had looked but I had not seen. I was guilty of "selective sight." In my heart I believed that I could cope with his ailments, but these new symptoms were indicative of depression and that was frightening to me. I didn't need a medical degree to know that this was a serious matter requiring prompt attention. He normally never would have acted this way. He was usually calm and could take everything in stride. How long had he been feeling so frightened? So depressed? I had asked him about depression from time to time before this, but he always had denied it. "Me? Depressed? Can't a man have an off-day without being accused of being depressed?

Tired? Yes! Overworked? Yes! Lost some weight? Yes, but what's so bad about that? Just don't nag me about it. Lu, you read too many health magazines."

This last outburst had taken place several weeks before, but now the sight of his pitiful countenance shook me to my roots. Where do we turn? What do we do? I couldn't allow him to see or feel the panic I was experiencing. I put my arms around my husband and held him as we rocked slowly back and forth. I spoke softly to him, assuring him that we'd get some help, because this was too complicated for us to handle on our own. I spoke with love and determination and Bob knew that together we'd cope with this too. We had faced other crises in our lives and now this was just an additional hurdle to surmount.

It was difficult for Bob to put his feelings into words, but he kept repeating the fact that he didn't want to be a burden on me, and he felt that our future was too bleak to contemplate. He knew he'd now have to take early retirement, and he felt that giving up his veterinary practice would be like ending his useful life. He took a deep breath and choked out the words, "Lu, I'm not good at anything anymore. I can't even make you happy in bed. I'm no longer a **man** and the more I try, the more I'm certain that I am almost impotent as well. Lu, you'd be better off without me."

"Aha," I said to myself. "At last he's starting to be honest about his feelings. He's been in denial for so long that this is a step in the right direction, but I'd better act quickly before he reverts to denial once again." Later that day when we were both calmer, I phoned a psychiatrist recommended by my best friend. Luckily, the doctor gave us an appointment for the end of the week.

Bob was reluctant to go because he couldn't see how merely talking to a psychiatrist would help. He found it difficult to describe his feelings and to reveal these private agonies to a stranger made him uneasy. As he put it, "Maybe I have a mental block about shrinks, but I'll give it a try–if you insist."

It was the best decision we could have made. After the first session, some of my husband's reticence faded. It took several visits before we started to see some improvement, but it was a learning experience for both of us. Dr. Dlin spoke with my husband while I waited in an outer office. Then he interviewed me, and in the last twenty minutes the three of us conversed. The doctor explained that it usually takes one to three sessions to establish a diagnosis and it's helpful to see the spouse of the patient in order to be provided with full background data. (Sometimes the patient is unable to report the symptoms with complete honesty.) Treatment is usually psychotherapy, but sometimes it is combined with medication. "Depression," Dr. Dlin told us, "is sometimes due to biological reasons and sometimes it's from external stimuli such as a major problem at work, medications or illness." We all concluded that Bob's Parkinson's disease and some of his medications were affecting his sexuality.

I wondered aloud why I had not seen depression's full impact for such a long time. I was usually quite sensitive to changes in my husband, yet I had failed to identify Bob's depressed state. I just thought he was getting irritable and unreasonable for no particular reason. I blamed it on overwork and aging, and thought he just needed a vacation. I had not understood the enormity of his mood swings.

We were told that depression comes on slowly and there can be a build-up over months or years (my feelings of guilt lessened a little with this information). Dr. Dlin told us that depression takes many forms. For example, a depressed person may:

1. **Work all of the time–pushing until exhaustion sets in**
2. **Avoid responsibility**
3. **Experience loss of energy**
4. **Experience loss of appetite**
5. **Become despondent**
6. **Be overly sad or cry easily**
7. **Have difficulty sleeping or stay in bed as a refuge**

We came away from that session convinced that the psychiatrist was right on target, and this gave Bob renewed confidence in his new doctor. During another session we learned that sexual dysfunction was often one of the early signs of depression. Bob and I exchanged knowing looks, and when we returned home we felt as if Dr. Dlin had somehow been an unseen observer in our bedroom. He had targeted symptoms such as:

1. **Withdrawal from social life**
2. **Withdrawal from sex**
3. **Withdrawal from a loving relationship**
4. **An inability for the patient to respond sexually**

Bob had experienced each of these symptoms, and it was now easier for him to reveal his anxieties. Trust had been established between us and the doctor, and that was a tremendous plus. Bob was comfortable talking with him and they conversed easily. We felt that we were getting the help we needed (I say "we" because Bob's depression affected both of us).

We also had a conference with my husband's neurologist, and he reviewed the medications and made a few changes because some of the drugs had an adverse effect on the libido. We had not thought about that, nor had we been told about it before this.

Dr. Dlin suggested that in order for my husband to overcome sexual dysfunction he had to be reassured that I was still interested in intimacy, even if it didn't end in intercourse. The emphasis was on improving our quality of life and the love we had for each other.

I was advised to put aside any inhibitions I might have had and focus on becoming a more imaginative sexual partner. Because of Bob's sexual frustrations it was up to me to try to rekindle his interest in sex and give him the encouragement he needed to engage in sexual intimacy. That made me think! What could I do to help my husband help himself? He needed to regain his self-esteem, to feel like my lover once again.

I knew I couldn't rush him into a situation that might have a discouraging effect upon him. We both knew that any anxiety about performance would always block true sexual intimacy. We were also aware that there would be episodes of absent ejaculation or reduced intensity of his ejaculation, and as seniors we should accept that as not being unusual. It was a challenge to balance what we knew intellectually with how we responded emotionally.

I had to cope with Bob's sexual dysfunction plus his depressed state of mind. I truthfully do not know if this depression was caused by his sexual problems or whether his sexual dysfunction was caused by his depression. It was imperative to slowly convince my husband that sexuality was not just penis-vagina-and-intercourse. All in due time. First we concentrated on loving closeness, gentle affection and trust. We shared feelings and sensations, then we moved on to pleasurable touching of one another. No passion, no lust; We simply moved cautiously and enjoyed the tenderness, caressing and fondling that brought us to shared pleasures. I was usually successful at this stage. I could wheedle or coax my mate into a better mood. Despite his many down periods I could tease him into responding to me. At times my hugs and kisses and snuggling made him smile. I could always go to him and say, "Sweetie, all I need is a hug. Do you have a big one for me? Make room on your lap for an old lady who loves you, and invite me to hop aboard." And I'd snuggle under his armpit for a few minutes of contentment.

I would remember Dr. Dlin's advice to me and toss my inhibitions aside, and at these times I'd flirt with my husband in a manner that made it clear that I was aiming to seduce him. He'd break into a smile and say, "I'm from Missouri." We'd laugh and I'd suggest that he hum the song called "The Stripper." (Every good act needs some background music.) Then I would go into a fake and exaggeratedly stagey version of a striptease–with the emphasis on tease. Not only would Bob hum the song, but he'd also clap his hands rhythmically in time to the music. Once I had disrobed, it was understood that I expected him to get into the act as well. Of course this bit of nonsense ended in laughter and increased desire, and once again I would hear the refrain that I treasured so "Lu, you're good for me!" I know that this is not for everyone; most people are too inhibited. But take the advice of a song that was popular in our youth and "let yourself go!"

You say you love me,
And you show it too
With thoughtful little
Things you do.
Oh! How I appreciate you!

CHAPTER 7
POSITIVE ATTITUDES

In the '90s the buzzword seems to be ATTI-TUDE. Attitude is the cue that will affect your sex life. We all can't be trim, slim, beautiful people with that "come hither" look, especially at our age. So it boils down to what signals you emit to your partner that you are interested in making love. Is sex a mechanical experience or is it innovative and enjoyable? Are you apprehensive with a defeatist attitude, and go about it with the feeling that "I'll try–but I'll fumble, and it will only end up as a frustration for both of us"?

Every Parkinson couple has frustrations! After a day of feeling grumpy and irritable, how can your partner be expected to come to bed with an "I'm ready" attitude toward sex? Set the stage for inti-macy long before you go to bed, or else it will be a complete turn-off. Sometimes a subtle hint about "pleasures to be had" will change your spouse's disposition for the remainder of the day, because it redirects the focus from one's problems to one's adventurous spirit between the sheets. Attitude! It declares, "Even with Parkinson's, I still desire you."

Years ago when my husband was first both-ered by short-lived erections, I felt guilty because I thought I wasn't doing enough to arouse him sexually. The more I tried, the less successful I was, and frustrations were quickly hampering both of us. Luckily, we were always able to speak honestly with each other. He assured me that I always turned him on and I had no need to feel guilty, but unfortunately his Parkinson's and the required medications often produced such a result. His attitude was: Today's was an unfortunate occurrence, who knows - maybe tomorrow it will be better.

Now every couple has a "love language" of their own—I believe this is universal. Bob called his penis Willie. He would say, "Sweetie, Willie is just getting cold." When he was dejected, he'd say it stood for Wee-Willie, and I'd tease him and say, "No, it stands for Willie-or-won't he." We were always able to laugh at and with each other.

After hearing "getting cold" once too often, the silly part of me took over. I found two pieces of felt, cut them to the appropriate size with pinking shears, stitched them together leaving one end open, and threaded thin blue satin ribbon through the top. I placed this beautifully wrapped gift upon his pillow, and called it his WILLIE WARMER. Bob looked at it, unbelieving. Then a huge smile broke across his face and he roared with laughter. When the sound died down, the spirit of my prank took over. He tossed the gift gently aside and said, "Love, you're good for me—come to me." I had diffused what could have been another tense situation by offering an upbeat attitude.

My husband and I shared a double bed. I felt loved and happy within his arms; he felt calm, protective and secure within our relationship. His Parkinson symptoms had escalated over the years and now his muscle spasms and restless sleep patterns were having a debilitating effect on both of us. Bob would be in and out of bed every hour and a half to two hours. Each time he thrashed around in bed I'd be aware of his movements and be semi-alert, anticipating his needs. It got to a point when the dark circles under my eyes made me look like a raccoon, and both of us went through the daily chores in slow motion.

I knew this had to stop, but how could I suggest separate beds to my husband? He'd feel rejected. His attitude was if you loved me you would not want to be apart from me. I wasn't pushing him out of my life—only my bed. How could I continue to cope with the stresses of caregiving if I constantly felt on the verge of collapse from lack of sleep? I tried explaining. I wheedled, I sweet-talked. All to no avail. He was adamant! His attitude wouldn't change. If I loved him, how could I take away this cherished part of his life? I prodded—he pulled back. I advanced my two-beds project, and he rejected the entire idea as a ludicrous and expensive experiment. It was a duel of desires.

At last, weary of my words, he agreed to purchase two identical double-sized beds for our room. He was still unhappy, I knew, but we had finally come to a joint decision and I was bound and determined to make it work. Too much was at stake! My womanly wiles had won. I made a concerted effort to let my husband know that I still loved him, and I would always love him, and he was welcome to share my bed any time he desired. That became a mutual invitation. We could still fall asleep in each other's arms, but he could leave my bed and toss and turn in his own bed without fear of awakening me. Bob soon found that it was now easier for him to sleep better because he had the entire width of his bed to himself, and he didn't have to concern himself about the spasms or jerking movements of his legs. He'd often be awakened by me in the early morning hours. I'd crawl into his bed and warm my cold feet against his toasty legs, snuggle against his body, plant a kiss upon his lips, and then we'd doze off contentedly for an extra hour until dawn. I'd make it my business to flirt with him and make him feel that I always desired him.

Bob liked to sleep nude because he found pajamas or nightshirts too binding when turning in bed. He also liked me to be nude beside him because he enjoyed the sensations my body gave him. Some evenings I'd purposely shower, powder, and don one of my sheer nighties before I slipped under the covers. Cue? Mood? Attitude?

"Why?" he'd ask me, grinning knowingly from ear to ear. My answer was always the same, "BECAUSE–It's a preview of coming attractions." Laughter followed.

I believe in the value of humor. My husband loved puns. We often relaxed in bed and enjoyed the give-and-take and teasing that accompanied a comfortable relationship. Bob would delight me with one of his groan-provoking puns and I would respond by one-upmanship. These horrible puns escalated until we shook with laughter and our bed rocked back and forth. But Bob would always get in the final pun. One night during a pun-fest I silenced him by declaring, "Hmmmmm, our bed's rocking from laughter now, but I remember when the bed shook, and bed slats crashed to the floor, for other reasons." I waited a moment for my declaration to sink in, then we laughed once more, and curled up in each other's arms. Beds were always important to us. They weren't just for sleeping.

Humor will often deflect a tense situation. I was told of a woman who was frustrated by her husband's lack of attention to her sexual needs. It seemed to her that he never wanted to have intercourse with her anymore. One night as he pulled back the bed covers he found his wife nude except for one item of clothing–crotchless panties. Above the cut-out section she had painted the words **enter here,** and then she had drawn a red arrow pointing downward to her pubic area. Who could have mistaken this message? A little creativity and a non-blaming attitude saved the night.

Couples who cope with disabilities are forever plagued by frustrations. I have found that with a solid marriage the disability actually brings the couple closer to each other. However, a disability within a rocky marriage tends to weaken the ties. The patient can either be grateful for the loving care received, or he can resent his loss of independence and respond to his mate's good intentions with a spiteful or unappreciative attitude. The healthy partner may feel a strong need to nurture and protect the mate who is chronically ill, or she may feel anger toward him for foisting the role of caretaker upon her. Anger and frustration do not have to be voiced to become apparent. It is seen in the set of the jaw, the tone of the retort, the forced smile, the slam of a door, or body language in general.

The aging and chronically ill continue to berate themselves for all the things they used to do so easily, and now find difficult or impossible. This is normal. The solution is to concentrate on the positive by undertaking tasks you are still able to master. It has been proved that patients with a positive attitude and the ability to laugh at life's foibles are the ones who have a better quality of life. Older people who value life and make the most of each day are the happiest of our senior citizens. The average lifespan has lengthened. Living to an older age is a privilege we've been granted. Even the chronically ill have good days. There are relief-filled hours within a truly bad day, for which we must be grateful.

Work on your attitude. Enjoy the pleasures of being touched, of being held or kissed, the playfulness and the deepened passions that we have learned along the way. Appreciate the loving relationships and count your blessings. Let your attitude become an affirmation of love and life!

You light my fire

And fill me with desire.

CHAPTER 8
THE TURN-ON

The brain is the most sexual organ in the body and controls the five senses that lead to our sexual pleasures. Sight, smell, touch, taste and sound are usually taken for granted. But they have the power to create the loving and exciting atmosphere we desire.

The brain enables us to fantasize and escape the humdrum or painful existence of our world. Through fantasy we can travel to far-off exotic places, control any situation and become the love-partner of anyone in the world. We can imagine ourselves young and slim or one of the beautiful people. Our imagination can make us strong and virile once again, healthy and handsome, with the most sought-after of the world's most seductive women. We can be masterful or submissive or assume any role the creative mind conjures up.

Memory can also help establish an atmosphere conducive to romance and be an inspiration for playful passion. Reminiscing about sexual prowess in the early years of marriage can serve as a starting point for sexier feelings and laughter. For example, the first hotel room that my husband and I shared gave us a wickedly free and sinful feeling. We arrived at the hotel after 10 p.m. with only a tote bag for our essentials. The clerk asked for our luggage and when we said we had none, his mouth twisted into a smirk while he shouted to the bellman, "No luggage!" The bellman took up the call and repeated, in an unnecessarily loud voice, "No luggage!" It seemed to reverberate across the hotel lobby. My husband's neck and face turned beet-red and I shifted nervously from foot to foot. Once we were in our assigned room we both exploded with laughter from the inference. Bob kept teasing me about being a wily wench and a sexy siren. After that unforgettable experience, all hotel rooms became a turn-on where formalities were abandoned, and we again assumed the roles of seducer and femme fatale.

Everyone creates new memories each day of our lives, but shared memories of past pleasures often have a stimulating effect upon our libido. Then our romantic fires are re-ignited.

Sexual appetite can be enhanced by our sense of sight. A man's desires may be increased by viewing his wife's full breasts because they produce thoughts of the delights of nuzzling his head upon their two soft "pillows." However, another man might be turned on by his wife's small breasts, assuring her that they are a "perfect mouthful." When he fondles them her erect nipples "stir his juices." Men may become aroused by the sight of a woman's ample hips swaying when she walks.

Or, a woman's tiny wiggle when she sits and crosses her legs can make his day.

Females are also sexually aroused by the sight of an attractive male. She may be turned on by his tanned body or the tight fit of his shorts or a bulging jock strap. The sight of his long fingers stroking her thigh can make a woman flush with anticipation. When she nibbles at his ear or throat and watches his heightened reactions, she knows they've both begun to throb sexually. Watching your partner's positive reaction to your overtures produces the "BIG-S": Supreme Sexual Satisfaction.

We can't really categorize the impact of our five senses on our desire for sex. The fragrance of a favorite perfume, body oil or lotion can create romantic images in our mind. The scent of fresh flowers from the garden can remind us of the times we lay together on the grass and enjoyed the hot kisses and cool breezes. The aroma of a man's pipe being smoked appeals to some women and brings to mind a truly masculine image of someone strong and protective. For some, the simple smell of the body is a complete turn-on. Any aroma that is a reminder of a sexual encounter can stimulate your senses.

Do you like to snuggle and cuddle? Does the warmth of your mate's body excite you? Do you enjoy rubbing your hand or face against the roughness of his beard or the tangle of hair upon his chest? Does a close embrace start you tingling? When your bodies rub against each other does it become a moment of arousal? This often happens when a couple dances to sensuous music. The words can have a special romantic meaning for the pair, or the rhythm may influence them to sway lovingly in each other's embrace. Music has always had the power to stir our emotions, from the rat-a-tat-tat of the earliest drums to the stirring sounds of the bugler; from the funeral's mournful dirge to the impassioned flamenco.

Music can set the mood for romance. For example, my husband was only a mediocre dancer, but he loved to hold me in his arms and sway to the music when we played our favorite "golden oldies." They brought back such romantic memories! He'd swirl and twirl me around and seize every opportunity to bend his body deeply over mine. With eyes half-closed, he'd hum softly, and occasionally he'd nibble at my ear. I'd feign surprise as he'd glide me from the den into the bedroom, dreamily continuing his off-key rendition of the song. Was it the sweetness of his kisses, the rhythmic movement of our bodies in unison, the reveries of past joys that made us so happy? The music, the dance, the close embrace–ah–romantic coupling then took the lead in our dance of love.

Our sounds can also be a powerful stimulant.

Whispered suggestions and messages actually increase our desires and guide our responses. Love-moans and groans convey meanings which need no further interpretation. We can progress from sweet, low, cooing and pet names to soft or rapid breathing, panting, or cries of rapture, and end with delight at the sounds both bodies make at culmination.

Top side,
  Down side,
Right side,
  Round side;
Together we will share the fun
  of merging, two becoming one.

CHAPTER 9
ENVIABLE POSITIONS

"Not my parents! Oh no! They're too old to have sex–to even be interested in having sex. It's not just their age. Remember that dad has Parkinson's disease, and he's got problems. I just can't imagine them doing it."

Sound familiar? I smiled knowingly and told the young woman that this was a common misconception. People of all ages, with and without physical disabilities, still have sexual feelings, urges, desires and yearning. She looked at me with disbelief, nodded her head and said, "Frankly, I can't picture that!"

This reminded me of days gone by when young pre-teens, who were newly aware of their bodies, were positive that their parents never did it. The very idea of this threw them into gales of laughter and nervous titters. One would say, "Yeah, but we're here, so they must have," and then they'd agree that IT probably happened only a couple of times when their parents were young, but not now because they're old.

Age and disability are not deterrents to feelings of sexuality. It's a personal matter. Some choose to pursue sexual activity. Others choose to veto the idea. There is another group who would like to be sexually adventurous but lack the knowledge or creativity required to accommodate to a disability. This is understandable. It requires a partner who is patient, encouraging, and who does not frustrate easily. Kathy, a young Parkinsonian, reminded me that in bed each partner is equal; they are no longer patient and caregiver.

Bob and I always thought of sex as fun and play. There were no pressures to perform. Our attitude? What happens, happens. If a new discovery gave us pleasure, that was a plus and something to be remembered. If not, there was always "tomorrow."

My husband was a tease. I always claimed that he taught me everything I knew about love and sex, and he claimed that I was the one who taught him. We were both correct. Oh, we were never exceptional lovers, nor were we "bedroom athletes," but our close and caring relationship warmed our hearts and it filled us with joy to reaffirm our love. This continued throughout our entire married life, including the sixteen years of coping with his Parkinson's disease.

If someone had asked me, "What was the nicest compliment your husband ever gave you?" my answer would have come quickly (in fact, I always smile when I think of it). He said, "After all these years you still turn me on." Now that is something

I'll never forget!

One of my great delights was to come into the bedroom and find that my husband had placed our pleasure pillow on the floor, and had propped it against the side of the bed. It was just an extra pillow kept for this special purpose. This was his non-verbal invitation, which relayed the message to me that he'd enjoy physical intimacy at that time. We found that when the pillow was placed under my hips it made it easier for him to enter me, and the changed angle, although slight, made it more comfortable and more pleasurable for both of us.

An application of a water-soluble lubricant such as K-Y jelly alleviated my vaginal dryness and helped him glide into me without causing discomfort for either of us. The lubricant felt icy-cold initially, so it was stroked on slowly to avoid the feeling of shock. Sometimes we both used it, depending upon the need. Boy Scout that he was, my husband was always prepared with a tube of lubricant and a clean handkerchief within easy reach on the night table–just in case.

As time went by and his Parkinsonism escalated, we found it necessary to experiment with other positions to accommodate his limitations. All it took was a little creativity and a lot of experimentation. We tossed away our inhibitions and recognized that this was an exciting challenge that we were both willing to tackle. Would it mean making love someplace other than our bedroom? A different time of the day or night? A variation of a position we had already found exciting? An assistive device? Just thinking about it was stimulating!

The usual position for most couples is the "missionary," where the woman lies on her back and her partner supports himself above her. The woman's legs can either be flexed, hooked around her lover's back, or her ankles can rest upon his shoulders. A lot depends upon mobility and stamina at this time. If he's not too agile, he might find this position hampering and difficult, because the man does most of the work.

One of the negatives about this position is that it often becomes uncomfortable if the male is much larger in stature than his partner. For some unexplained reason, I have found that many tall men often tend to select small women for a partner. Does this bring out the protective instinct in him? The missionary position will often put too much weight upon women who feel as if they are being crushed but find it is an awkward time to complain.

We had to discover positions that would allow my husband freedom of movement, but would not put too much stress on his arm or leg muscles. We wished to avoid stress and cramping of his neck muscles too. We sought positions that were comfortable, practical, and which often had me assuming the more active role.

A favorite position was to nestle like spoons, each of us on our side, and he was able to enter the vagina from the rear. Clitoral stimulation added to the intensity of arousal for me and excitement for him. A variation of this position was for each of us to lie on-side, facing each other, but intercourse this way had me providing most of the movement.

Still another "resting position" that is easy on the male is for him to lie on his side facing his partner, while his loved one is on her back with flexed legs resting over his thighs. This sounds complicated, but is really not. And it allows the woman to move her body into different angles. This heightens arousal for both lovers.

I truly enjoyed having my husband lie on his back with me astride him. His hands were then free to caress my body as my hands brought him pleasure. I was in control of the tempo he desired, and which we both wished to establish, and this brought about fantastic arousal for each of us.

A Parkinson couple approached me hesitantly. They wanted to tell me about their favorite sexual position but were a little uneasy about broaching the subject. Once the wife and I began to talk, the husband looked less embarrassed.

The wife was the Parkinsonian. She said that the only reason they agreed to the interview was that, despite her Parkinson dyskinesia, they had a beautiful and satisfying sex life. They wanted to share their success in order to help other couples who might be having sexual problems.

They described the position that worked best for them. She sits on her husband's lap facing him, their legs spread apart. This position allows them to make eye contact, is comfortable for both partners and causes no physical stress for either of them. Arousal can be enhanced by mutual fondling.

The husband said that he prefers to sit in a straight-backed chair, but that is just a matter of personal choice. As they departed, he whispered to me, "If we come up with other successful positions we'll share them with you. Actually, we'll be glad to work on it."

There is another option for couples who are having sexual difficulties because of a soft erection. This is a common occurrence and many couples are discouraged because of it. The solution is for the female to initiate the "stuffing technique." She sits astride her partner and slowly and tenderly stuffs his flaccid penis into her vagina, whose warm and moist atmosphere helps stimulate it. If she tightens her pubococcygeus muscle (PC) at the same time, it may help to improve or prolong his erection. **Warning:** Insert the penis with a gentle stroking and stuffing motion, a little at a time, and be careful that your fingernails do not dig into it or scrape his testicles. Another suggestion is to take this action seriously because if you laugh, his penis will be forced out by the contraction.

You will learn to identify and tighten the PC muscle by doing the KEGEL EXERCISES devised by Dr. Arnold Kegel. Although they are designed to improve bladder control, these exercises also strengthen the PC muscle for added vaginal control. My gynecologist gives his patients a page of instructions introducing these exercises. They're easy to do and can be practiced anywhere.

I am certain that if you experiment and allow your creative instincts to take over, frustrations will decrease and your sexual pleasures will increase. If you share feelings of tenderness, love and affection it will help overcome the negatives. Although all these suggestions may not lead to full penetration or even completion of intercourse, they will certainly bring about a flurry of activity and a flush of pleasure. Sometimes the pleasures are far more important than the accomplishment. Think of all this exercise you've had–the calories you've burned–the elevated heart rate–and the atmosphere of excitement. Wow! You'll agree it was worth it.

Fingers playing joyfully
Caressing self with care,
Sensitive to body's needs
  Of which I am aware
  –And do not wish to share.

CHAPTER 10
THE TENDER TOUCH

Masturbation used to be considered a dirty word that was never said openly, and was relegated to uneasy whispers and raised eyebrows by our elders. People who are now in their sixties, seventies and older were reared by parents with Victorian ideas about sex. When I asked my daughter if she remembered any myths about masturbation she quickly replied, "Mom, those myths were a generational thing." Her answer startled me at first, but then I realized that she was correct.

My generation rarely questioned its elders, and blindly accepted their statements as fact. Boys were told that regular masturbation would ultimately lead to blindness; some were warned that eventually it would result in insanity. One gentleman laughed when he told me that when he was young his mother assured him that if he continued to masturbate, the fluid would leave his spine and he would eventually become paralyzed. Teenagers examined their hands on a daily basis because they were threatened with stories of masturbation resulting in hairy palms. Guiltily they refrained from this practice as much as possible because they didn't want anyone to know they did it, as evidenced by palms turning hairy. Boys were instructed to keep their hands out of their trouser pockets because parents feared that their sons would be secretly fondling their genitals, and that was unacceptable behavior.

We now know that masturbation is a marvelous release from tension and can be practiced by women as well as men. Men are usually very frank about having masturbated for most of their lives, and they treat it as they would any normal biological function. Women, however, are usually reluctant to discuss the subject. What holds them back? Perhaps feelings of shyness, a lack of instruction, or feeling too embarrassed to discuss it with anyone. One woman said, "I'd feel funny touching myself THERE." Several women I interviewed thought it was disgusting and could never get themselves to caress their own bodies, but there were many other women who highly recommended it. Some said that they had never masturbated but they were willing to try it. Others needed to be reassured that masturbation is not just for the young, but is a good outlet for the elderly and the disabled as well.

Attitudes must change with the decades. It's exciting to have sex with a partner, but when no partner is available it can be just as rewarding an experience to pleasure yourself. Statistically, women outlive men. Widows continue to have sexual feelings long after their spouse is gone, and eligible men their age or older are in scarce supply or are impotent. Therefore, we find that as we age, masturbation plays a larger role in the sexual practices of seniors. Widowers generally have no hang-ups and pleasure themselves without guilt.

Widows and widowers often complain about their sleepless nights. It's not unusual to hear them declare, "I tossed and turned all night long and couldn't get comfortable. I finally got out of bed at 4 a.m. and read until the sun came up." If they had released some of their tensions by masturbating, they would have been more relaxed and able to enjoy a restful sleep.

Couples unable to complete the sex act can still find pleasure in self-gratification or in mutual masturbation. This doesn't mean that there is something wrong with their marriage. Some women become annoyed or have hurt feelings when they see a spouse fingering his penis. The wife feels that something has gone out of their marriage and wonders if she's not sexy enough to satisfy him. She asks herself why he has to do this. Why couldn't he ask her for sex instead of whacking at himself like an adolescent? Their relationship is still the same. Nothing is wrong. It's just that each person has different needs and frequencies of desire. There are many wives who are frustrated by their husband's impotence, and the women find that self-gratification makes them feel like sexual beings, feminine and desirable.

Masturbation should be a source of pleasure. You are the one who is in control. You can prolong the exquisite sensations or you can slowly build toward arousal. Orgasm can be achieved through manual stimulation and often can be enhanced by the use of fantasy. If you decide to enjoy this form of sexual pleasure, set the mood as if you were going to have a sexual encounter with a partner. Never attempt to set a schedule for regular periods of masturbation. Indulge only when you are in the mood. Tune in to your own feelings. Be comfortable with your body's responses. Experiment until you find the areas that create the greatest feelings of arousal. You may desire soft music and muted lighting in your bedroom, or wish to use aromatic oils or lotions. Another suggestion is to luxuriate in a bathtub filled with warm, sudsy water, allowing the slippery soap film to help you glide your hands over your body. It's a sensuous way to discover your reactions to breast and genital stimulation at your own pace. There's no need to hurry. Savor the delights of the moment. Playful fingers can gently massage the area around the clitoris, or light pressure can be applied to this area. You are in charge of your own body and self-arousal usually leads to orgasm. You'll find that you will emerge from this experience with a feeling of renewal.

Males find it easier to accept masturbation, and

are less inhibited about it. The head of the penis and the underside of the shaft are the most sensitive areas for the male. The corona, which is the ridge at the back of the penis-head is also an area of intense feeling when it is fondled. You can vary the sensations by using a dry hand or fingers that have been lubricated with K-Y jelly (lubricants tend to increase a person's sensitivity). Some men enjoy the gentle manipulation of the scrotum.

Masturbation can be a solo or a shared experience, depending upon your desire. A joyous variation is mutual masturbation. Older couples, and those who are limited by disabilities, often find complete satisfaction in watching their partner become aroused. At times the man will watch or assist the woman until she climaxes, and this will become an erotic turn-on for him. She can either stimulate him manually, or he can pleasure himself while she is the observer. At times the male must educate his partner in the act of manual stimulation. He must impress upon her that time is needed to savor the sensations that are brought on by a mixture of slow and fast strokes. A man must communicate his wants or needs at that particular stage of arousal. My husband loved to whisper suggestions that would guide my hands or change my tempo. At one point he smiled with pleasure and whispered, "Lu, you play me like the finest musical instrument–slowly, gently, building to a crescendo. I should have your hands insured by Lloyds of London." Happiness was etched upon his face. We were in tune with each other.

The couple can enjoy self-gratification, each tending to his or her own needs but enjoying the pleasures simultaneously, or they can masturbate each other. Vocalization at this point should be a part of the release. It's also a turn-on to hear the pleasure-moans of your partner and it adds heightened stimulus to the act.

Some people find that sexual arousal can be intensified by the use of vibrators, using various pressures, and alternating slow and feathery-light touches with faster or firmer contact. Sometimes it is advisable to stop for a few moments to let the arousal subside a bit, and then shift your playfulness into a different direction until climax or orgasm has been achieved. Older men need not ejaculate each time in order to experience orgasm. Try creative love overtures and see how your areas of sensitivity can be enhanced.

Pink tongue
Soft, yet strong,
Flicking
Licking
Slipping
Sliding
Curling
Swirling
Probing
Caressing
Ending
in
Ecstasy

CHAPTER 11
RENEWED PLEASURES

When dealing with sexuality, masturbation and oral sex are two controversial subjects. "Baby Boomers" readily accept both as normal functions, but persons two and three decades older have lived most of their lives feeling that these activities are to be frowned upon.

Enlightenment about oral sex has given many couples a new lease on life. Sexual dysfunction often leads to heartbreaking depression, and a man who is impotent has to deal with his loss of performance, his crumbling ego and the frustration of his mate. How many times have they eagerly tried to make love, only to have all activity come to a halt when his penis cannot become erect. He mumbles apologies and half-promises that we'll try again later. But she knows and he knows that each fiasco makes it more and more difficult, and it builds to a terrible letdown. She may turn away from him physically or emotionally, or lash out with uncontrolled anger because of her frustration and disappointment. If she tries to console him he may misconstrue this as pity and retreat in stony silence to his "I'm no longer worth a damn as a man" mood. He silently yearns for sexual gratification for each of them and despises the changes that are taking place in their lives.

Many couples have found that oral sex is the answer to this problem. It brings new excitement and fulfillment to their union. If loss of an erection is a problem, oral sex provides the pleasure, stimulation and release without the fear of failure. If intercourse is painful for the woman, she may welcome the new experience. Couples no longer have to deal with a sex life focused on penis-into-vagina performance. Creativity enhances their lovemaking. The tongue, lips and mouth are now thought of as sexual organs that can be sensitive as well as stimulating. Oral sex can be used as a preliminary or, as we experience aging and disability, it can become the "main event." It is less tiring for both partners and requires little physical stamina. Success is practically guaranteed.

What is involved? Cunnilingus is the stimulation of a woman's genital area by her partner's mouth or tongue. Fellatio is the oral stimulation of the penis.

Cleanliness should be the primary concern. If the body is washed before intimacy then there is no offensive taste or odor. A shared shower or bath, or having your partner bathe you or wash your hair, can be wonderful foreplay. Even if your thoughts are not of a sexual nature, you owe it to yourself and your spouse to adhere to a strict regimen of cleanliness. In fact, after my daily shower my husband used to go into a fake lament. "Didn't your mama ever teach you how to dry yourself?" he'd complain with a grin. "You're still half-wet!" Then he'd proceed to towel-dry the droplets on my back and shoulders, working down to my legs with loving care. This became a fun ritual. The faint perfume of my soap and shampoo, my skin that had turned pink from the needle-like spray of hot water pelting my body, even my shiny face, became a turn-on for him.

Reactions to oral sex cover a wide range. A silver-haired gentleman and his wife admitted quite frankly that it gave them more pleasure than they ever thought possible at their age. They're very open with each other as to their desires, and she coyly said, "You know, it makes us feel young again and we actually look forward to these romantic interludes." He squeezed her hand in agreement. I smiled as I caught the glint in their eyes that was an affirmation of their joy in each other.

I had a telephone interview with a woman who felt she'd be less inhibited in discussing sexuality with me if we were not face-to-face. She confessed that years ago her husband had asked her for oral sex, and she declined because she felt it was dirty and she felt she couldn't do it. He never again requested anything other than the missionary position. She told me that they had fewer and fewer sexual encounters and eventually terminated that part of their relationship. Now that she had read more about the subject, she said that she regretted all the years that were lost. I told her that there was no need to feel guilty or abnormal for not wanting oral sex. It was a personal decision and there should never be any pressure for anyone to do something that was distasteful to them. She continued, "My four daughters would probably say there is nothing wrong with this activity. They're more open about sex. Perhaps if I were younger and of a different generation's mind-set I'd have been able to make my husband's last years happier this way."

Oral love-play lends itself to experimentation. The tongue is covered with tiny little nerve endings. A tongue running playfully over your lover's ear, neck or nipples stimulates arousal. The same is true for a kiss on the small of the back or upon the genital area. Don't hurry! Take your time and allow your lips and tongue to probe and explore. Discover ways to bring pleasure to each other.

There are many kinds of kisses that bring a rush of excitement: quick and fluttery kisses the length of the penis shaft, slow and gentle kisses enclosing the tip of the penis, long and deeper kisses back and forth, and sometimes merely flicking the tongue on sensitive areas.

Any of these can bring a person to orgasm. Soft breath gently blowing patterns across the clitoris or vaginal area, genital kisses and a probing tongue can arouse a woman to such a degree that she can experience multiple orgasms.

Some women are reluctant to perform oral stimulation because they have an urgent gag reflex and are afraid of taking the penis into their mouth. If this is the case, simply kiss the tip of the penis because the ridge, or corona, is the most sensitive area for the male and that's enough to provide heightened sexual stimulation. I've also been told that some women don't want their mate to ejaculate into their mouth. For some it's due to the gag reflex; other women just feel uncomfortable with the idea (the taste is not unpleasant and nothing will happen if semen is accidentally swallowed). The solution is to tell your partner to alert you when he is almost at the point-of-no-return, and then pull away and allow him to ejaculate into a clean tissue or handkerchief, which you have ready for this purpose. Once again I stress the need for good communication. This may now be a time when you really appreciate snuggling contentedly in each other's arms, relaxed and happy.

Tell your lover what pleased you, what you dislike, what you'd like to try. Remember that you may be wary of doing something today but may feel more adventuresome the next time. Or perhaps the joy you've found today may suggest another variation to be tried in the future–an exciting thought to be shared. It has to be something you both want to do, not something you've been pressured into doing. Continue to be open to suggestion, be creative, relax and enjoy.

Devices
Are
Not
Vices

CHAPTER 12
TO THE RESCUE

Do you believe advertisements and testimonials that promise a one hundred percent success rate in increasing the size of your erection? Or guaranteeing that if you use their product you WILL have an erection? Are you aching to be rescued from your emotionally charged sexual despair?

Children's literature stresses the thrilling rescue of damsels in distress. Some books describe brave police officers or firefighters who rush to the rescue of unfortunate people whose lives have been imperiled. We have grown up fully expecting to be rescued by good Samaritans and daring heroic measures.

Adults send up fervent prayers. We bargain with God to aid us in coping with chronic illness. We plead with doctors to cure us. Sometimes we elevate physicians to god-like status and create expectations that can never be fulfilled.

Chapter 5, "The Fear of Impotence," describes erectile dysfunction and promises that there is help for this condition. Impotence is a problem that affects the male and his partner. Speak openly about it with each other. It's certainly not something that you can hide.

The decision to try alternatives must be jointly made–a choice made by partners. There are various aids and devices available to help you cope with impotence. Are both of you comfortable with the idea? You'll need patience and understanding.

When you seek professional help and treatment, make certain that you have utmost confidence in the urologist. The first step is assessment: discovering whether or not your problem is psychological or physical. In order to evaluate your dysfunction the physician will probably require the following information or diagnostic tests:

1. complete medical and sexual history
2. urological examination
3. blood and urine tests
4. penile blood pressure and sensation evaluation
5. sleep monitoring
6. X-ray of your penile veins/arteries

Once the diagnosis of impotence is confirmed, your urologist will be able to offer a wide spectrum of possible suggestions, including assistive devices and medical/surgical procedures. Solutions depend upon how important it is to you and your partner, and other factors including your overall health, age or pre-existing chronic conditions. Your health insurance may also influence your choices. Remember that you are not in this by yourself– your mate shares your frustrations and can help make the decision that is appropriate for both of you. An excellent Medical Essay Supplement of the Mayo Clinic Health Letter, February 1993, states:

"Only a few years ago, doctors generally thought that about 90 percent of impotence was psychological. Now they realize that 50 to 75 percent of impotence is caused by physical problems. There is a wide range of treatments. Keep in mind that the success of any treatment depends, in part, on open communication between partners in a close, supportive relationship. Here are some options:

1. **Psychological therapy** - Many impotence problems can be solved simply by you and your partner understanding the normal changes of aging and adapting to them. For help in this process, your doctor may recommend counseling by a qualified psychiatrist, psychologist or therapist who specializes in the treatment of sexual problems.

2. **Hormone adjustment** - Is testosterone a magic potion for impotence? No. Although testosterone supplementation is used in rare instances, its effectiveness for aging men experiencing a normal, gradual decline in testosterone is doubtful.

3. **Vascular surgery** - Doctors sometimes can surgically correct impotence caused by a de-

creased blood flow to the penis. However, this bypass procedure is appropriate in only a small number, less than two percent, of young men who have impotence problems. The long-term success of this surgery is too often disappointing.

4. **Vacuum device** - Currently one of the most common treatments for impotence, this device consists of a hollow, plastic cylinder that fits over your flaccid penis. With the device in place, you attach a hand-pump to draw air out of the cylinder. The vacuum created draws blood into your penis, creating an erection.

   Once your penis is erect, you slip an elastic ring over the cylinder onto the base of your penis. For intercourse, you remove the cylinder from your penis. The ring maintains your erection by reducing blood flow out of your penis. Because side effects of improper use can damage the penis, you should use this device under your doctor's care.

5. **Self-injection** - Penile injection therapy is another option. It involves injecting a medication directly into your penis. One or more drugs (papaverine, phentolamine and prostaglandin El) are used. The injection is nearly painless, and produces a more natu-

ral erection than a vacuum device or an implant.

6. **Penile implants** - If other treatments fail or are unsatisfactory, a surgical implant is an alternative. Implants consist of one or two silicone or polyurethane cylinders that are surgically placed inside your penis. Implants are not the perfect solution. Mayo experts say there is a 10 to 15 percent chance an implant will malfunction within five years, but the problem almost always can be corrected. Many men will find the procedure worthwhile.

   There are two major types of implants: one uses malleable rods and the other uses inflatable cylinders. Malleable rods remain erect, although they can be bent close to your body for concealment. Because there are no working parts, malfunctions are rare.

   Inflatable devices consist of one or two inflatable cylinders, a finger-activated pump and an internal reservoir, which stores the fluid used to inflate the tubes. All components–the cylinders, pump and reservoir–are implanted within the penis, scrotum and lower abdomen. These devices produce more "natural" erections.

7. **Medications** - Neurotransmitters are chemi-

cals in your brain and nerves that help relay messages. Nitric oxide is now recognized as one of the most important of these chemicals for stimulating an erection. Unfortunately there is as yet no practical way to administer nitric oxide for treatment of impotence. Other drugs have not proved effective."*

A man may shudder at the thought of injections in his penis. In reality, the pain is slight and lasts only a few moments. The discomfort must be weighed against the benefits. An erection that is produced by penile injection usually has a duration of one-half to three-quarters of an hour. It should also be noted that all of these procedures have risks associated with them.

Many couples do not want to handle impotence with the use of a pump, cylinder or injection. They are wary of these choices, and opt for oral sex and/or masturbation to satisfy their sexual appetite. They no longer require penetration to fulfill their sexual needs. The elderly enjoy the extra time it takes for arousal. Some find this alternative to be a more satisfying experience than the hasty and frantic

*Reprinted from February 1993 MAYO CLINIC HEALTH LETTER ©1993 Mayo Foundation for Medical Education and Research, Rochester, Minnesota 55905. Reprinted by permission©

coupling of their youth. They prefer the latter years' slow and sensual dance of love. Love sessions may be fewer in number but they are certainly more appreciated.

Some men and women find that vibrators come to the rescue and add to their enjoyment of sex. Battery operated, vibrators can be used by men or women—alone or with a partner. Older women often turn color at the mere mention of the words vibrator or dildo. They would not want to be seen in an "Adult Gift Shop."

One friend quipped, "The only way I'd go into one of those places would be if I was decked out in a big hat with a heavy veil and wearing dark glasses. I'd worry about being seen there." Another woman said, "Oh my! Just think of all we missed— my husband and I!"

We each handle our sexual practices in our own way. There are many choices available. Select the solution, activity or device that gives you and your partner the greatest pleasure and peace of mind.

A WIDOW'S LAMENT

I see him now upon the bed.
He'd turned to stone from foot to head.
His color–granite–stays with me!
With eyes closed, I still can see
This statue–the man I love
Whose spirit rose to God above.
My loss was great–it shook me so...
He died quickly, and it was hard to know
Just what to do.
They told me, "Dear, your husband's gone!
Breathe deeply...try...you must hold on."
My last words to him were "I love you!"
He'd whispered softly, "Love you, too."
It's two years since that awful night
I've cried, I've coped, with the wrenching fright
Of what to do and how to do it–
Where to turn–so much to learn!
"You're strong" I hear the couples say–
(Don't know why friends have dropped away.)
Are they reminded of what lies ahead?
Their future lives hanging by God's fine thread?
I force a smile upon my face
Knowing...widowhood is no disgrace.

CHAPTER 13
SENIOR SINGLES: SURVIVORS

The last years of my husband's life were happy and productive. His death was sudden, totally unexpected. We had always talked about death as we did about life; we joked and laughed, yet Bob always tried to prepare me for this eventuality.

We bought a loose-leaf notebook and devoted a page each to pertinent information about funerals, insurance, investments, the car's upkeep and other important topics. It was a guidebook for the uninformed. This was serious business, but we laughingly decided that, because I was forever misplacing things, we'd put this information in a bright-red binder that would almost scream "Here I am–I'm easy to find."

Over the years, we updated the information to keep everything current. I'd ask Bob, "Are you preparing me for widowhood?" One part of me knew this was the truth, but a greater part of me preferred denial: Bob was doing fine–It wouldn't happen soon–We weren't ready–There's lots of time before I'd have to face the "Big D" of death.

There were lighter moments, of course. My husband loved to say that I was unique, but he pronounced it "u-nee-que." One day he observed, "You know, Lu, on your tombstone I'll have them inscribe:

> Here lies Lu
> She's "u-nee-que"
> She's not like me
> And she's not like you."

I giggled and said, "Nah, you won't do that. They charge for each letter and you're too cheap." Quick as a flash he retorted, "You're right! I'll settle for R.I.P."

I always thought I would predecease my husband. This stemmed from the fact that in 1970 I was diagnosed with a life-threatening illness for which there is no known cause or cure. I'd tease my husband about his becoming a widower and I'd say, "Bob, the night of my burial some enterprising woman will come to the door with a container of chicken soup in one hand and an apple pie in the other. She'll smile invitingly and say that they need a fourth for bridge, and damn it, you'll go." We spoke about death and dying as if it were the most natural thing in the world, which of course it is.

When I joined the huge sorority of Singles, it was an eye-opener and a heart-breaker at the same time. We all know that unmarried women outnumber unmarried men. Widows and divorcées are dubbed "the singles" and they're slowly pushed aside by married friends. They're relegated to afternoon lunches, telephone calls, shopping or all-female functions. No longer are they invited to participate in couples' dinner parties because there must be a man for every woman present, and male-female numbers have to be kept even. A mundane entertainment such as a movie requires that couples go with other couples, singles with singles. I have been told, "Oh, we saw the best movie on Saturday night. You must take yourself to see it."

Widowers, however, are always in demand socially, no matter how dull or uninteresting they are. Their physical limitations are overlooked as well. Women cluck like mother hens over any single male and they are always looking out for his welfare. Widowers rarely remain unattached for long. Single women know that widowers are used to being waited on and catered to, so they pounce upon the newly bereaved man and offer the comfort and warmth of female companionship, as well as home-cooked meals. Before he knows it he's hooked!

Married women view widowed women as a threat to their happiness and a reminder of the frailty of life's thread. No one wants to be reminded that they, too, may one day swell the ranks of the elderly Singles.

Each person handles bereavement in his or her own way. It is said that the normal period of grieving is usually two years. Of course that varies from person to person. It's a period of intense frustration and vulnerability. And whatever can go wrong will do so.

For example, when my husband died there was a mix-up with Social Security. They had me listed as deceased and my husband alive. Consequently, they halted my benefits. The last check they had issued me was removed from my bank account. Their actions affected my Medicare as well. I had to appear in person at a Social Security office with documentation proving my identity, and I had to swear out an affidavit that I was alive and the true Lucille Carlton.

My nerves were on edge and my eyes constantly puddled. Each decision assumed enormous proportions. I tried not to panic, and my bright-red loose-leaf notebook became my Bible. When Bob died I was perceived to have lost my identity. It took a long time, but with help and a network of support, I was able to gather strength each day and became my own person, secure in my decisions. After two long years I was able to announce to my children, "I still miss dad, I think of him each day, I talk to him when I need help, and now I can truthfully say I am back on track. I'm comfortable living alone."

"I've made new friends, and I'm now self-reliant. Dad was a good teacher; he'd be proud of me." Yes, my husband groomed me for widowhood.

There are people who are bitter about the death of their spouse. They lament that life will never be the same. They're right! It's never the same; there are constant changes in your living patterns. Men and women who argued and bickered with each other all the time now describe their "dear departed" in glowing terms that practically elevate their mate to sainthood. Yes, they miss their spouse. They miss the quarrels and they miss the interaction. It's lonely when you have no one to answer you. Silence is deafening and sound takes on a new importance.

Men and women without partners rate loneliness as the number one frustration. They crave companionship. Some actively seek relationships with the opposite sex. Others sit back and wait for an introduction by mutual friends. A woman told me that her advanced age didn't matter; she didn't feel feminine without a man. On the other hand, another woman declared that she wasn't looking for a second husband because, in her opinion, "All these old men want is a nurse or a purse." I've watched a man who took no interest in his personal appearance during the year following his wife's death, suddenly turn into a Beau Brummel when his interest was sparked by a diminutive female in his age group. Each time he took her to dinner his appearance was impeccable and his step was livelier. It was a joy to watch him exude happiness.

I've spoken with many Singles across the country and their desires are similar. Humans want to feel needed and appreciated. Older men and women can be as giddy as young lovers in the company of the opposite sex. When one-half of the pair dies, the other person still has a life to live, hopes and desires to fulfill, and stirrings of sensuality to acknowledge. It's when you finally realize that you are indeed a whole person, deserving more out of life than just living in the past, that you know you can finally make a new life for yourself.

Does this life include a member of the opposite sex? That's a personal choice. Many Singles would welcome an escort to the theater, a concert, a lecture or another social event. Repartee between the sexes is usually perceived as more stimulating and discussions of current events and politics more challenging than similar single-sex encounters. Dining alone is not really dining–it's usually bolting food rapidly just to get the meal finished, with little or no interest in the quality or preparation of the food. When a meal is shared with someone, it becomes a time of conversation and shared enjoyment, eaten at a slower and more relaxed pace, and sweetened by appreciation.

Do we need a member of the opposite sex in order to be happy? The answer is **yes** and **no**. Happiness is found within your own person, and you have to be in touch with your own inner-peace to achieve this goal. However, another person can contribute to your feelings of well-being. Senior Singles miss being touched, hugged, comforted and caressed. Some crave sexual fulfillment while others merely desire companionship.

A few women will discuss second-pairings in the abstract. They deny personal interest in the opposite sex but offer opinions about others who are intimately involved. Statements emerge such as, "He's so unappealing. What does she see in him? I guess all she's looking for is the proper plumbing." One widow said, "How could I undress in front of a man? I'd feel so embarrassed." It's a very personal and emotional experience to open your body to the intimacy of physical closeness. It requires trust and caring on the part of both partners. Thoughts tumble out one after another: Will he compare me to his first wife? Will thoughts of my dead husband make me feel disloyal? Why am I frightened? Do I fear disappointment? Can I set limits for my new partner? Will I be baring my soul once again? Questions and more questions, with only tentative answers.

Several years ago, I found that the husband of an acquaintance of mine had to be placed in a nursing home. His Alzheimer's symptoms had escalated to a point where she could no longer care for him without help. She worked in an office each day and visited her husband at the home at dinner time so she could feed him. Her guilt was assuaged because this way she was still taking care of him. An elderly gentleman visited his wife there on a daily basis for the same reason. The two caregivers began to talk, to commiserate with each other, and to lend support. They soon stopped for a cup of coffee before they went their separate ways, and then this led to shared dinners several times a week. They continued their visits to the home as part of their routine, but romance between the two blossomed. The sad part is that they became "Widow and Widower of the Living," which involved dealing with myriad feelings of guilt. I won't go into the moral issues involved, but each survivor has a right to love and to be loved.

There are senior Singles who travel together or set up housekeeping arrangements with shared expenses. This is a creation of the times in which we live. Other Singles feel they would be disloyal to their deceased spouse if they embarked upon another intimate relationship. Feelings of guilt gnaw at your gut. What will people think? How will children react to a parent's new "pairing"? Will there be resentment? Will there be acceptance?

I remember a night a year or so before Bob died. It was after a particularly delicious session of intimacy that my husband held me tightly in his arms, stroked my hair gently and lovingly, and said, "Honey, before I die I think I'll write a letter of recommendation to your second husband. You've given me so much happiness." I snuggled closer, but in my heart I knew there would never be another husband; God had already granted me the best.

What are your thoughts? Tell me, please,
    Would you?
    Could you?
    Should you?

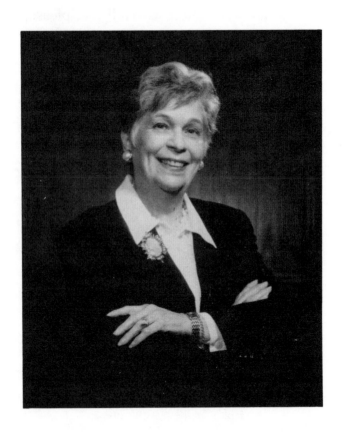

Lucille Carlton, educator and lecturer, writes a column, "Straight From the Heart" for the NPF Parkinson Report. With her husband, Bob, she co-authored, "Courage Behind the Mask; Coping with Parkinson's Disease," prior to his death in 1991. She is a graduate of Pennsylvania State University and has her masters degree in art from Temple University. The mother of three daughters, she resides in suburban Philadelphia.

If you have questions pertaining to problems of everyday life confronted by PD patients or caregivers, write to:

Lucille Carlton
c/o The National Parkinson Foundation, Inc.
1501 NW 9th Avenue
Miami, FL 33136

RESOURCE DIRECTORY

Printed information is available from the following organizations upon request:

ALZHEIMER'S ASSOCIATION
919 N. Michigan Avenue, Suite 1000
Chicago, IL 60611

AMERICAN ASSOCIATION OF
GERIATRIC PSYCHIATRY
P.O. Box 376A
Greenbelt, MD 20768

AMERICAN ASSOCIATION FOR
MARRIAGE AND FAMILY THERAPY
10th Floor
1100 17th Street
Washington, DC 20036

AMERICAN ASSOCIATION OF SEX EDUCATORS,
COUNSELORS AND THERAPISTS (AASECT)
435 N. Michigan Avenue, Suite 1717
Chicago, IL 60611

AMERICAN COLLEGE OF OBSTETRICIANS
AND GYNECOLOGISTS
409 12th Street, SW Washington, DC 20024

AMERICAN HEART ASSOCIATION
7320 Greenville Avenue
Dallas, TX 75231
(Local chapters found in many communities.)

AMERICAN PARKINSON'S DISEASE ASSOCIATION
60 Bay Street, Suite 401
Staten Island, NY 10301

ARTHRITIS FOUNDATION
1314 Spring Street, NW
Atlanta, GA 30309

CHILDREN OF AGING PARENTS
Woodbourne Office Campus
1609 Woodbourne Road, Suite 302A
Levittown, PA 19057

DEPRESSION AWARENESS, RECOGNITION, AND
TREATMENT (D/ART)
National Institute of Mental Health
D/ART Public Inquiries
5600 Fishers Lane, Room 15C-05
Rockville, MD 20857

This office can answer questions about drug ap-
proval process, drug reactions, and other issues con-
cerning new or approved medications.

HIP (HELP FOR INCONTINENT PEOPLE)
P.O. Box 544
Union, SC 29379

IMPOTENCE INFORMATION CENTER
AMERICAN MEDICAL SYSTEMS
P.O. Box 9
Minneapolis, MN 55440

MARRIAGE COUNCIL OF PHILADELPHIA
4025 Chestnut Street
Philadelphia, PA 19104

NATIONAL ALLIANCE FOR MENTALLY ILL
2101 Wilson Blvd., Suite 302
Arlington, VA 22201

NATIONAL INSTITUTE ON AGING
Public Information Office
9000 Rockville Pike
Building 31, Room 5C27
Bethesda, MD 20892

NATIONAL PARKINSON FOUNDATION
1501 NW 9th Avenue
Miami, FL 33136

NATIONAL WOMEN'S HEALTH NETWORK
1325 G Street, NW
Washington, DC 20005

PARKINSON DISEASE FOUNDATION
COLUMBIA-PRESBYTERIAN MEDICAL CENTER
650 West 168th Street
New York, NY 10032

SEX INFORMATION AND EDUCATION COUNCIL
OF THE U.S. (SIECUS)
130 West 42nd Street, Suite 2500
New York, NY 10036

UNITED PARKINSON FOUNDATION
833 W. Washington Blvd.
Chicago, IL 60607

For additional copies of "Sex, Love, and Chronic Illness" contact the National Parkinson Foundation, 1501 N.W. 9th Avenue, Miami, Florida 33136. Phone: 1-800-327-4545.

$13.95 (including postage and handling)

Checks, money order, Visa or Mastercard

Proceeds to be used for Parkinson research